How to use this journal

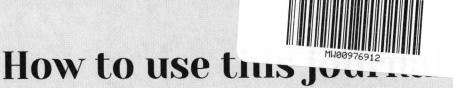
- Date: Keeping track of the date allows you to better track your habits on a daily basis. It can also serve as a reminder of your progress.

- Positivity: It is important to enter into this challenge with a positive mindset. Not only will it make it easier/more enjoyable, it will also help you to continue doing these exercises. Each week has a positive quote for you to meditate on. Every day, read this quote aloud to yourself. Speak life over yourself, your family, your situation. Proclaim them!

- Notes: Every day has a blank "notes" section. Use this space to write anything extra about your day: what good things happened to you, what negative things happened, what stood out to you in what you read and/or listened to, etc.

- Compliment: Every day, write down five things that you achieved and/or like about yourself. Reminding yourself of these things (or new things) daily help keep the enemy and his lies from penetrating your mind and spirit.

- Goals: Every week, strive to take the necessary steps to reach a set goal that you have for yourself. This can be physically, mentally, spiritually, financially... there is no right or wrong goal. Just write one down and work towards it.

- Schedule: Our bodies thrive on schedules. Keeping (to the best of your ability) a routine schedule can have lasting positive effects on your health, mentally and physically.

- Breathe: If you miss something on the list for the day, don't stress out about it. Recognize it, own it, and grow from it, striving to do better the next day. It takes about 10 weeks for something to become a habit, so by the end of this journey, you will have many healthy habits to build your life on.

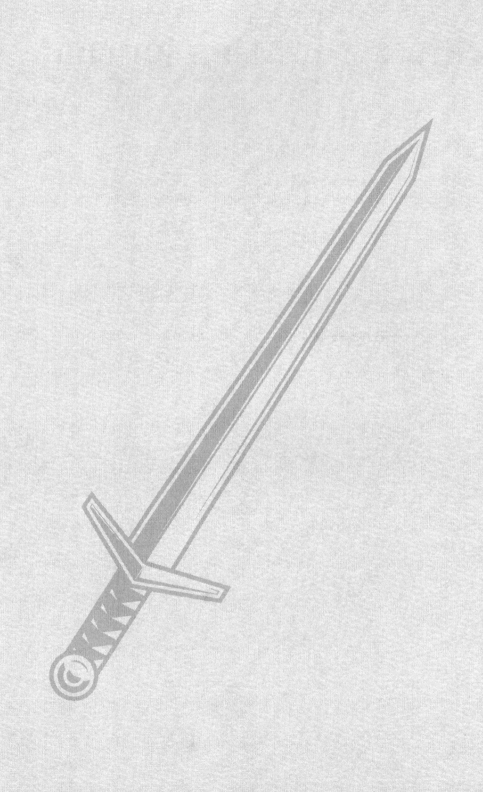

WEEKLY PLANNER

Week One

MONDAY

TUESDAY

WEDNESDAY

THURSDAY

FRIDAY

SATURDAY

SUNDAY

BEDTIME FOR THE WEEK:

DID I GO TO CHURCH?
☐ Yes   ☐ No

IF SO, WAS I LATE?
☐ Yes   ☐ No

GOAL FOR THE FUTURE:

DAYS I WILL STUDY FOR IT:

WEEKLY POSITIVE QUOTE:

I remain confident of this, I will see the goodness of the Lord in the land of the living. Wait for the Lord; be strong and take heart and wait for the Lord.

~Psalm 27:13-14

Day 1

DID I?

Eat healthy?
Yes   No

Eat when I wasn't hungry?
Yes   No

Work out?
Yes   No
If yes, what did I do?
_____

Walk/Run one mile?
Yes   No

Read 15 pages/chapters?
Yes   No
If yes, what did I read?
_____

Pray 15 minutes?
Yes   No

Eat fruit/vegetables?
Yes   No

Listen to a Christian Podcast?
Yes   No
If yes, what did I listen to?
_____

Rest without napping?
Yes   No

Five things I did good or like about myself today:

1. _____
2. _____
3. _____
4. _____
5. _____

One thing I could do better: _____

How can I achieve it? _____

_____

NOTES

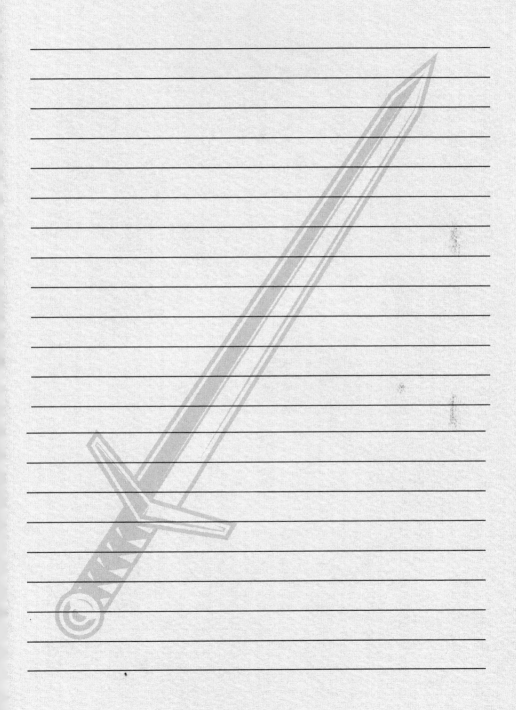

Day 2

DID I?

Eat healthy?
Yes   No

Eat when I
wasn't hungry?
Yes   No

Work out?
Yes   No
If yes, what did I do?
_____

Walk/Run one mile?
Yes   No

Read 15 pages/chapters?
Yes   No
If yes, what did I read?

_____

Pray 15 minutes?
Yes
No

Eat fruit/vegetables?
Yes   No

Listen to a Christian
Podcast?
Yes   No
If yes, what did I listen to?
_____

Rest without napping?
Yes   No

Five things I did good or like about myself today:

1._____
2._____
3._____
4._____
5._____

One thing I could do better: _____

How can I achieve it?   _____

_____

NOTES

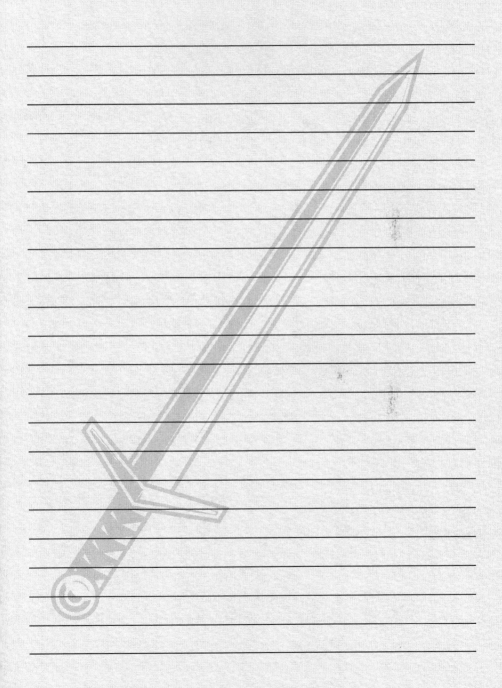

Day 3

DID I?

Eat healthy?
Yes   No

Eat when I
wasn't hungry?
Yes   No

Work out?
Yes   No
If yes, what did I do?
_____

Walk/Run one mile?
Yes   No

Read 15 pages/chapters?
Yes   No
If yes, what did I read?
_____

Pray 15 minutes?
Yes   No

Eat fruit/vegetables?
Yes   No

Listen to a Christian
Podcast?
Yes   No
If yes, what did I listen to?
_____

Rest without napping?
Yes   No

Five things I did good or like about myself today:

1._____
2._____
3._____
4._____
5._____

One thing I could do better: _____

How can I achieve it?   _____

_____

NOTES

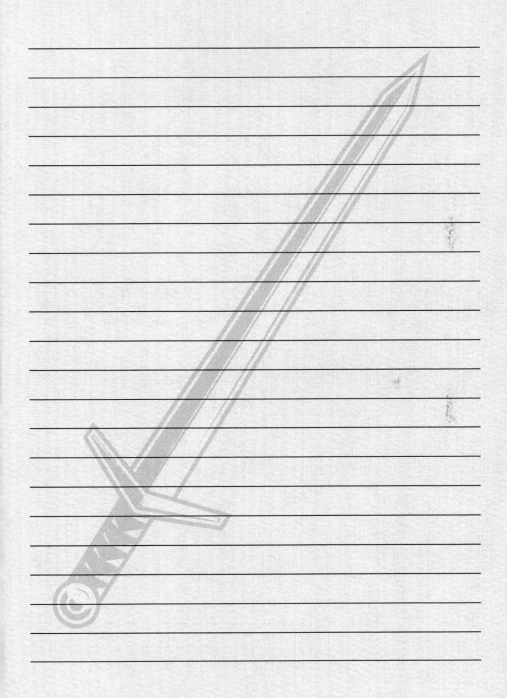

Day 4

DID I?

Eat healthy?
Yes   No

Eat when I wasn't hungry?
Yes   No

Work out?
Yes   No
If yes, what did I do?
_____

Walk/Run one mile?
Yes   No

Read 15 pages/chapters?
Yes   No
If yes, what did I read?
_____

Pray 15 minutes?
Yes   No

Eat fruit/vegetables?
Yes   No

Listen to a Christian Podcast?
Yes   No
If yes, what did I listen to?
_____

Rest without napping?
Yes   No

Five things I did good or like about myself today:

1. _____
2. _____
3. _____
4. _____
5. _____

One thing I could do better: _____

How can I achieve it? _____
_____

NOTES

Day 5

DID I?

Eat healthy?
Yes   No

Eat when I wasn't hungry?
Yes   No

Work out?
Yes   No
If yes, what did I do?
_____

Walk/Run one mile?
Yes   No

Read 15 pages/chapters?
Yes   No
If yes, what did I read?
_____

Pray 15 minutes?
Yes   No

Eat fruit/vegetables?
Yes   No

Listen to a Christian Podcast?
Yes   No
If yes, what did I listen to?
_____

Rest without napping?
Yes   No

Five things I did good or like about myself today:

1. _____
2. _____
3. _____
4. _____
5. _____

One thing I could do better: _____

How can I achieve it? _____

_____

NOTES

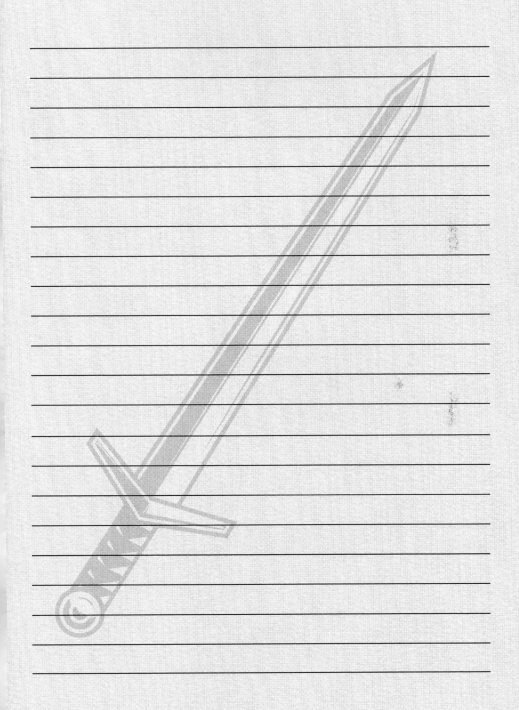

Day 6

DID I?

Eat healthy?
Yes   No

Eat when I
wasn't hungry?
Yes   No

Work out?
Yes   No
If yes, what did I do?
_____

Walk/Run one mile?
Yes   No

Read 15 pages/chapters?
Yes   No
If yes, what did I read?
_____

Pray 15 minutes?
Yes   No

Eat fruit/vegetables?
Yes   No

Listen to a Christian
Podcast?
Yes   No
If yes, what did I listen to?
_____

Rest without napping?
Yes   No

Five things I did good or like about myself today:

1. _____
2. _____
3. _____
4. _____
5. _____

One thing I could do better: _____

How can I achieve it? _____

_____

NOTES

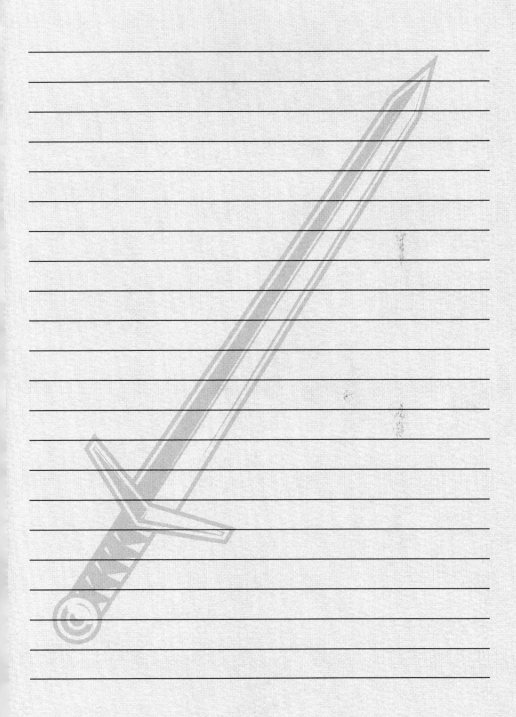

Day 7

DID I?

Eat healthy?
Yes   No

Eat when I wasn't hungry?
Yes   No

Work out?
Yes   No
If yes, what did I do?
_____

Walk/Run one mile?
Yes   No

Read 15 pages/chapters?
Yes   No
If yes, what did I read?
_____

Pray 15 minutes?
Yes   No

Eat fruit/vegetables?
Yes   No

Listen to a Christian Podcast?
Yes   No
If yes, what did I listen to?
_____

Rest without napping?
Yes   No

Five things I did good or like about myself today:

1. _____
2. _____
3. _____
4. _____
5. _____

One thing I could do better: _____

How can I achieve it? _____

_____

NOTES

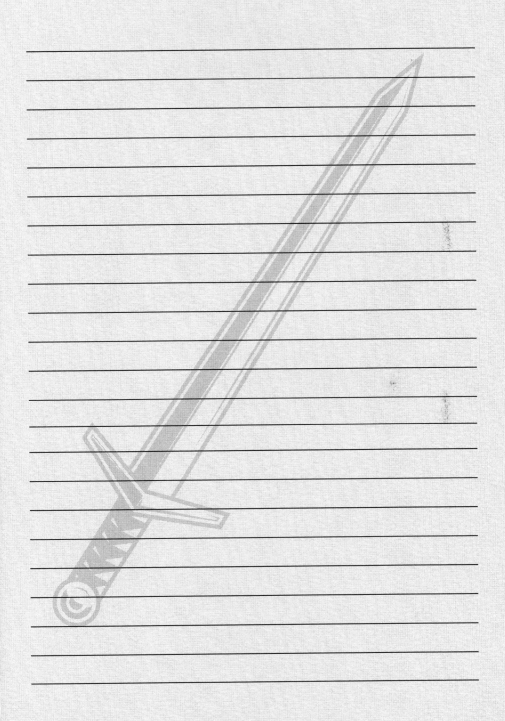

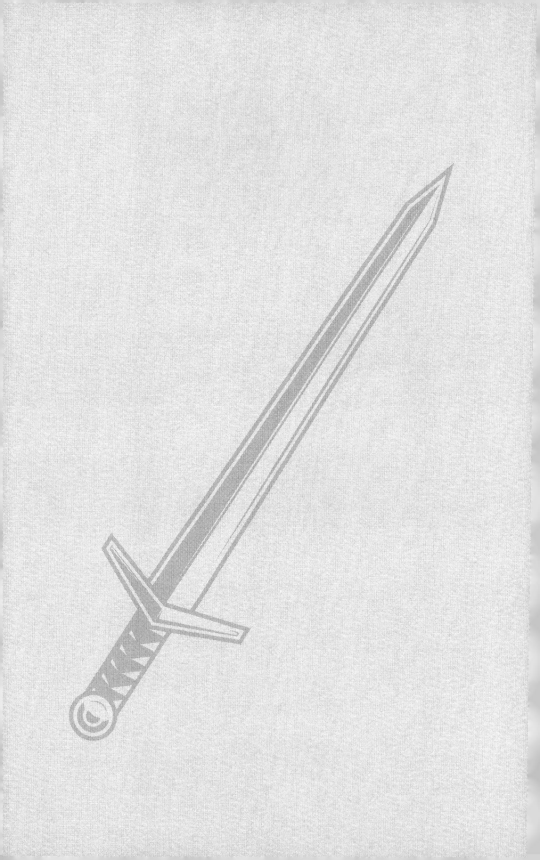

WEEKLY PLANNER

Week Two

MONDAY

TUESDAY

WEDNESDAY

THURSDAY

FRIDAY

SATURDAY

SUNDAY

BEDTIME FOR THE WEEK:

DID I GO TO CHURCH?

☐ Yes ☐ No

IF SO, WAS I LATE?

☐ Yes ☐ No

GOAL FOR THE FUTURE:

DAYS I WILL STUDY FOR IT:

WEEKLY POSITIVE QUOTE:

Keep this Book of the Law always on your lips; meditate on it day and night, so that you may be careful to do everything written in it. Then you will be prosperous and successful. Have I not commanded you? Be strong and courageous. Do not be afraid; do not be discouraged, for the LORD your God will be with you wherever you go.

- Joshua 1:8-9

Day 1

DID I?

Eat healthy?
Yes   No

Eat when I wasn't hungry?
Yes   No

Work out?
Yes   No
If yes, what did I do?
_____

Walk/Run one mile?
Yes   No

Read 15 pages/chapters?
Yes   No
If yes, what did I read?
_____

Pray 15 minutes?
Yes   No

Eat fruit/vegetables?
Yes   No

Listen to a Christian Podcast?
Yes   No
If yes, what did I listen to?
_____

Rest without napping?
Yes   No

Five things I did good or like about myself today:

1._____
2._____
3._____
4._____
5._____

One thing I could do better: _____

How can I achieve it? _____

_____

NOTES

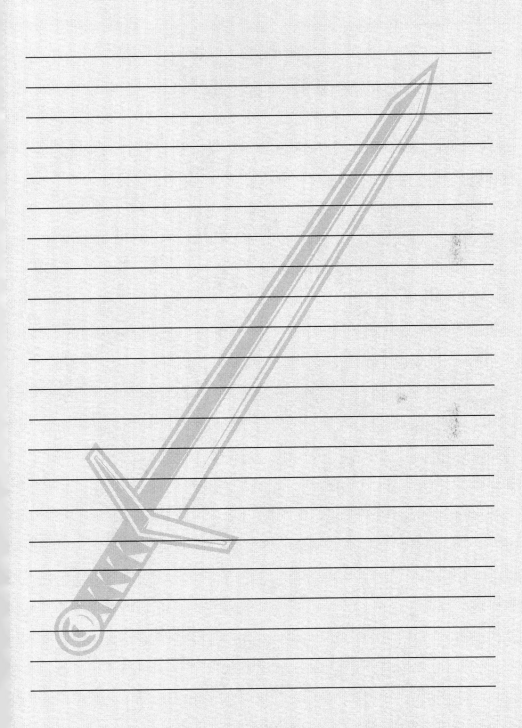

Day 2

DID I?

Eat healthy?
Yes   No

Eat when I
wasn't hungry?
Yes   No

Work out?
Yes   No
If yes, what did I do?
_____

Walk/Run one mile?
Yes   No

Read 15 pages/chapters?
Yes   No
If yes, what did I read?
_____

Pray 15 minutes?
Yes   No

Eat fruit/vegetables?
Yes   No

Listen to a Christian
Podcast?
Yes   No
If yes, what did I listen to?
_____

Rest without napping?
Yes   No

Five things I did good or like about myself today:

1. _____
2. _____
3. _____
4. _____
5. _____

One thing I could do better: _____

How can I achieve it? _____
_____

NOTES

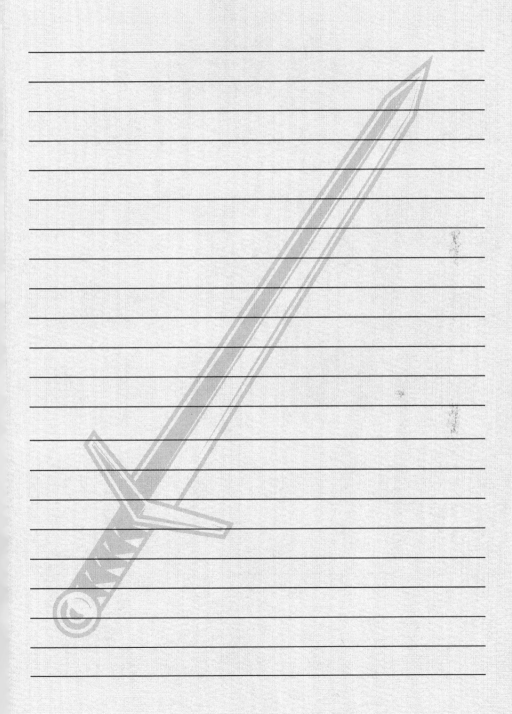

Day 3

DID I?

Eat healthy?
Yes   No

Eat when I wasn't hungry?
Yes   No

Work out?
Yes   No
If yes, what did I do?
_____

Walk/Run one mile?
Yes   No

Read 15 pages/chapters?
Yes   No
If yes, what did I read?
_____

Pray 15 minutes?
Yes   No

Eat fruit/vegetables?
Yes   No

Listen to a Christian Podcast?
Yes   No
If yes, what did I listen to?
_____

Rest without napping?
Yes   No

Five things I did good or like about myself today:

1. _____
2. _____
3. _____
4. _____
5. _____

One thing I could do better: _____

How can I achieve it? _____
_____

NOTES

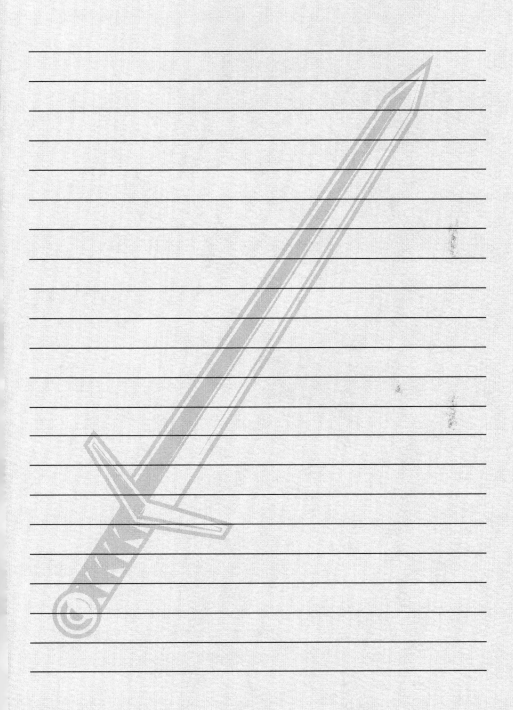

Day 4

DID I?

Eat healthy?
Yes   No

Eat when I wasn't hungry?
Yes   No

Work out?
Yes   No
If yes, what did I do?
_____

Walk/Run one mile?
Yes   No

Read 15 pages/chapters?
Yes   No
If yes, what did I read?
_____

Pray 15 minutes?
Yes   No

Eat fruit/vegetables?
Yes   No

Listen to a Christian Podcast?
Yes   No
If yes, what did I listen to?
_____

Rest without napping?
Yes   No

Five things I did good or like about myself today:

1._____
2._____
3._____
4._____
5._____

One thing I could do better: _____

How can I achieve it? _____
_____

NOTES

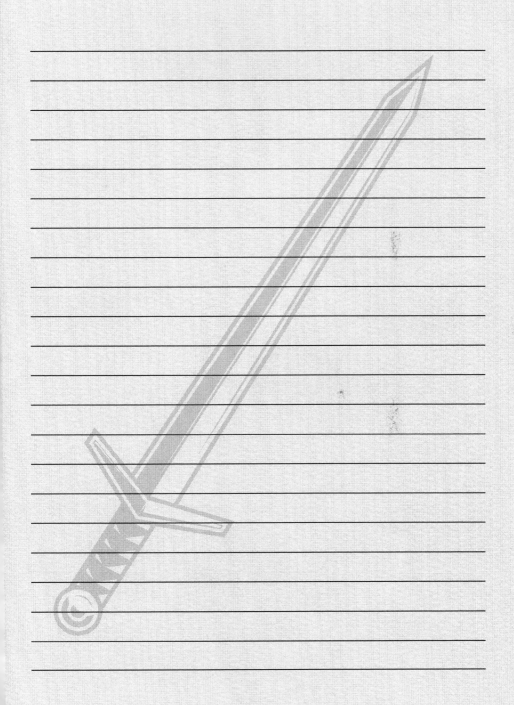

Day 5

DID I?

Eat healthy?
Yes   No

Eat when I wasn't hungry?
Yes   No

Work out?
Yes   No
If yes, what did I do?
_____

Walk/Run one mile?
Yes   No

Read 15 pages/chapters?
Yes   No
If yes, what did I read?
_____

Pray 15 minutes?
Yes   No

Eat fruit/vegetables?
Yes   No

Listen to a Christian Podcast?
Yes   No
If yes, what did I listen to?
_____

Rest without napping?
Yes   No

Five things I did good or like about myself today:

1. _____
2. _____
3. _____
4. _____
5. _____

One thing I could do better: _____

How can I achieve it? _____

_____

NOTES

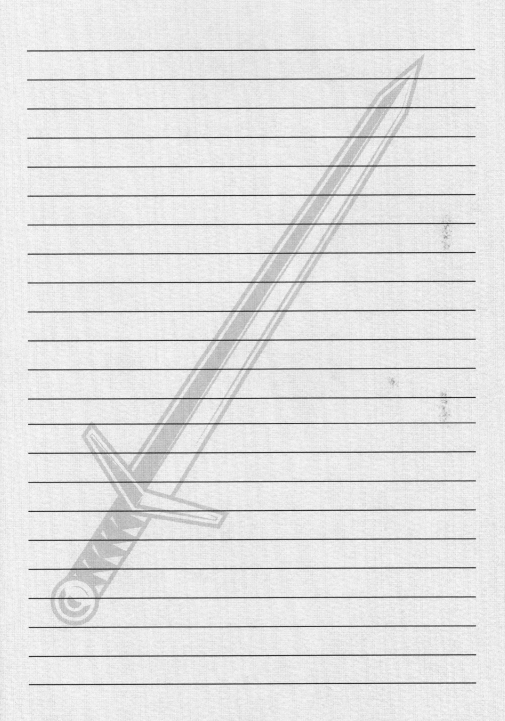

Day 6

DID I?

Eat healthy?
Yes   No

Eat when I wasn't hungry?
Yes   No

Work out?
Yes   No
If yes, what did I do?
_____

Walk/Run one mile?
Yes   No

Read 15 pages/chapters?
Yes   No
If yes, what did I read?
_____

Pray 15 minutes?
Yes   No

Eat fruit/vegetables?
Yes   No

Listen to a Christian Podcast?
Yes   No
If yes, what did I listen to?
_____

Rest without napping?
Yes   No

Five things I did good or like about myself today:

1. _____
2. _____
3. _____
4. _____
5. _____

One thing I could do better: _____

How can I achieve it? _____

_____

NOTES

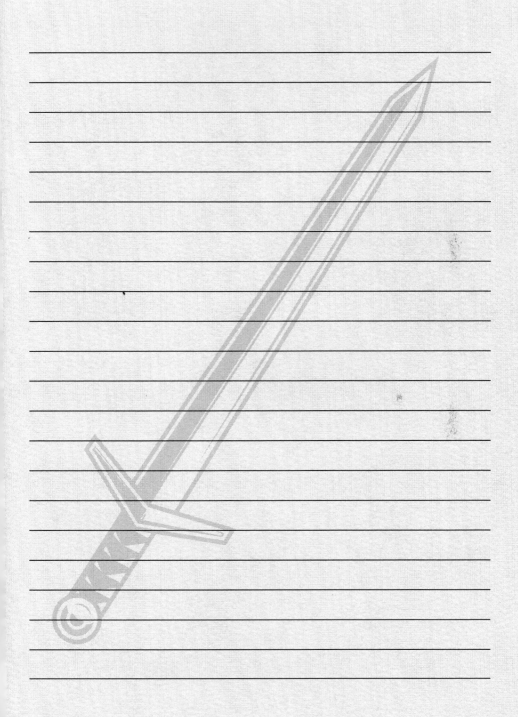

Day 7

DID I?

Eat healthy?
Yes   No

Eat when I wasn't hungry?
Yes   No

Work out?
Yes   No
If yes, what did I do?
_____

Walk/Run one mile?
Yes   No

Read 15 pages/chapters?
Yes   No
If yes, what did I read?
_____

Pray 15 minutes?
Yes   No

Eat fruit/vegetables?
Yes   No

Listen to a Christian Podcast?
Yes   No
If yes, what did I listen to?
_____

Rest without napping?
Yes   No

Five things I did good or like about myself today:

1. _____
2. _____
3. _____
4. _____
5. _____

One thing I could do better: _____

How can I achieve it? _____
_____

NOTES

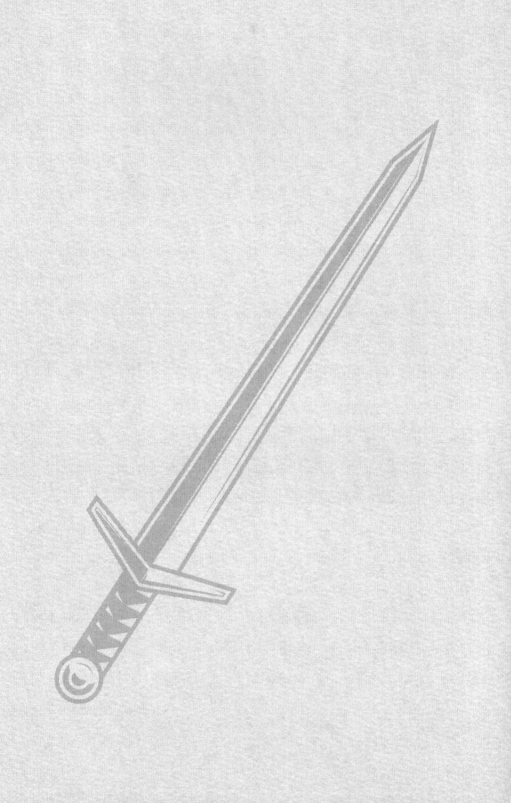

WEEKLY PLANNER

Week Three

MONDAY

TUESDAY

WEDNESDAY

THURSDAY

FRIDAY

SATURDAY

SUNDAY

BEDTIME FOR THE WEEK:

DID I GO TO CHURCH?
☐ Yes   ☐ No

IF SO, WAS I LATE?
☐ Yes   ☐ No

GOAL FOR THE FUTURE:

DAYS I WILL STUDY FOR IT:

WEEKLY POSITIVE QUOTE:

For the life of every living thing is in his hand,
and the breath of every human being.

-Job 12:10

Day 1

DID I?

Eat healthy?
Yes   No

Eat when I wasn't hungry?
Yes   No

Work out?
Yes   No
If yes, what did I do?
_____

Walk/Run one mile?
Yes   No

Read 15 pages/chapters?
Yes   No
If yes, what did I read?
_____

Pray 15 minutes?
Yes   No

Eat fruit/vegetables?
Yes   No

Listen to a Christian Podcast?
Yes   No
If yes, what did I listen to?
_____

Rest without napping?
Yes   No

Five things I did good or like about myself today:

1._____
2._____
3._____
4._____
5._____

One thing I could do better: _____

How can I achieve it?   _____

_____

NOTES

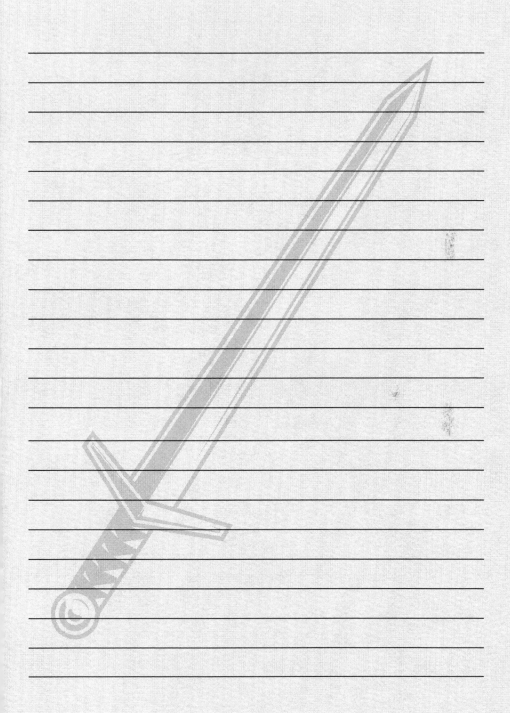

Day 2

DATE: /   /

DID I?

Eat healthy?
Yes   No

Eat when I
wasn't hungry?
Yes   No

Work out?
Yes   No
If yes, what did I do?
_____

Walk/Run one mile?
Yes   No

Read 15 pages/chapters?
Yes   No
If yes, what did I read?
_____

Pray 15 minutes?
Yes   No

Eat fruit/vegetables?
Yes   No

Listen to a Christian
Podcast?
Yes   No
If yes, what did I listen to?
_____

Rest without napping?
Yes   No

Five things I did good or like about myself today:

1._____
2._____
3._____
4._____
5._____

One thing I could do better:

_____

How can I achieve it?

_____

_____

NOTES

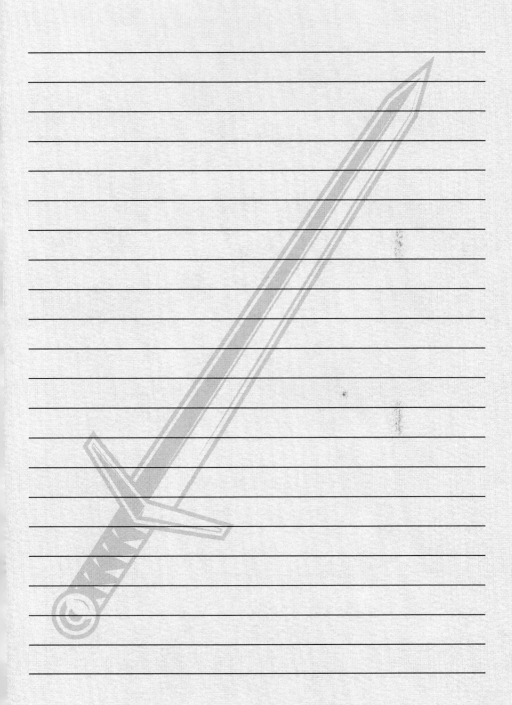

Day 3

DATE: / /

DID I?

Eat healthy?
Yes   No

Eat when I wasn't hungry?
Yes   No

Work out?
Yes   No
If yes, what did I do?
_____

Walk/Run one mile?
Yes   No

Read 15 pages/chapters?
Yes   No
If yes, what did I read?
_____

Pray 15 minutes?
Yes   No

Eat fruit/vegetables?
Yes   No

Listen to a Christian Podcast?
Yes   No
If yes, what did I listen to?
_____

Rest without napping?
Yes   No

Five things I did good or like about myself today:

1._____
2._____
3._____
4._____
5._____

One thing I could do better: _____

How can I achieve it? _____

_____

NOTES

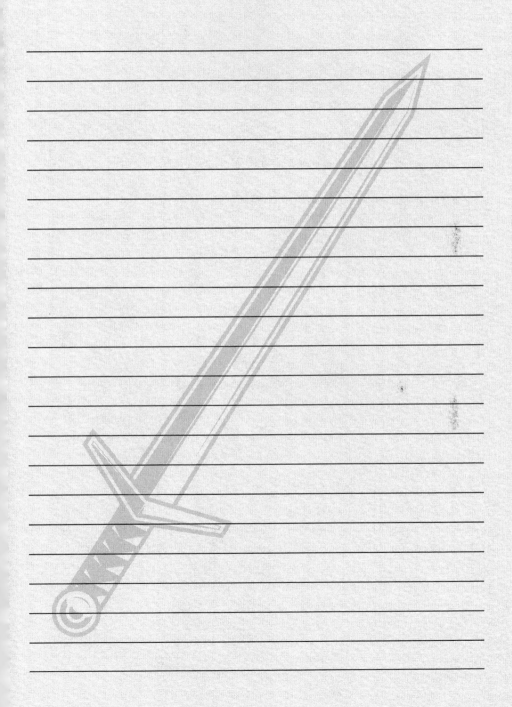

Day 4

DID I?

Eat healthy?
Yes   No

Eat when I wasn't hungry?
Yes   No

Work out?
Yes   No
If yes, what did I do?
_____

Walk/Run one mile?
Yes   No

Read 15 pages/chapters?
Yes   No
If yes, what did I read?
_____

Pray 15 minutes?
Yes   No

Eat fruit/vegetables?
Yes   No

Listen to a Christian Podcast?
Yes   No
If yes, what did I listen to?
_____

Rest without napping?
Yes   No

Five things I did good or like about myself today:

1._____
2._____
3._____
4._____
5._____

One thing I could do better: _____

How can I achieve it? _____

_____

NOTES

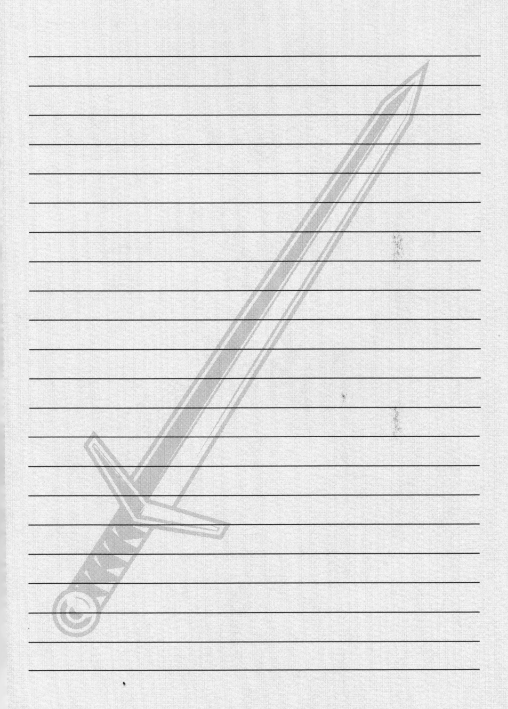

Day 5

DID I?

Eat healthy?
Yes   No

Eat when I wasn't hungry?
Yes   No

Work out?
Yes   No
If yes, what did I do?
_____

Walk/Run one mile?
Yes   No

Read 15 pages/chapters?
Yes   No
If yes, what did I read?
_____

Pray 15 minutes?
Yes   No

Eat fruit/vegetables?
Yes   No

Listen to a Christian Podcast?
Yes   No
If yes, what did I listen to?
_____

Rest without napping?
Yes   No

Five things I did good or like about myself today:

1. _____
2. _____
3. _____
4. _____
5. _____

One thing I could do better: _____

How can I achieve it? _____

_____

NOTES

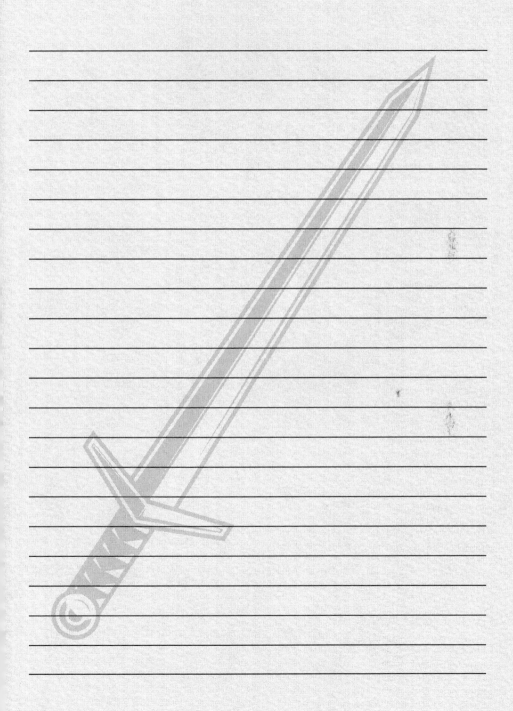

Day 6

DID I?

Eat healthy?
Yes   No

Eat when I wasn't hungry?
Yes   No

Work out?
Yes   No
If yes, what did I do?
_____

Walk/Run one mile?
Yes   No

Read 15 pages/chapters?
Yes   No
If yes, what did I read?
_____

Pray 15 minutes?
Yes   No

Eat fruit/vegetables?
Yes   No

Listen to a Christian Podcast?
Yes   No
If yes, what did I listen to?
_____

Rest without napping?
Yes   No

Five things I did good or like about myself today:

1._____
2._____
3._____
4._____
5._____

One thing I could do better:

How can I achieve it?

_____

_____

NOTES

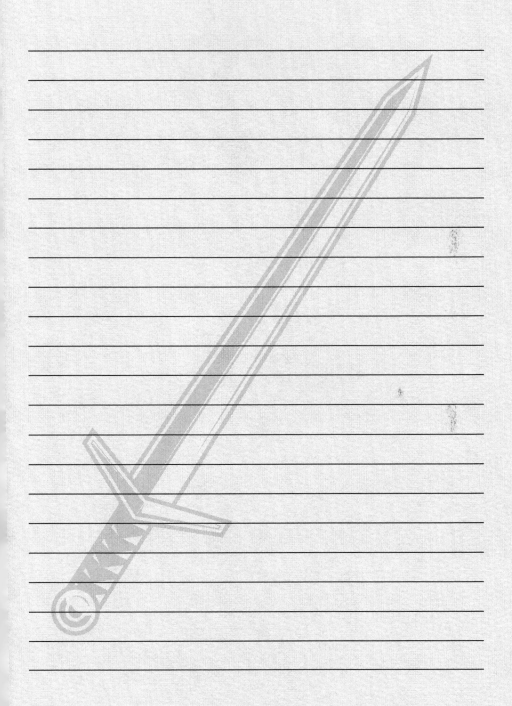

Day 7

DATE: / /

DID I?

Eat healthy?
Yes   No

Eat when I wasn't hungry?
Yes   No

Work out?
Yes   No
If yes, what did I do?
_____

Walk/Run one mile?
Yes   No

Read 15 pages/chapters?
Yes   No
If yes, what did I read?
_____

Pray 15 minutes?
Yes   No

Eat fruit/vegetables?
Yes   No

Listen to a Christian Podcast?
Yes   No
If yes, what did I listen to?
_____

Rest without napping?
Yes   No

Five things I did good or like about myself today:

1. _____
2. _____
3. _____
4. _____
5. _____

One thing I could do better:
_____

How can I achieve it?
_____
_____

NOTES

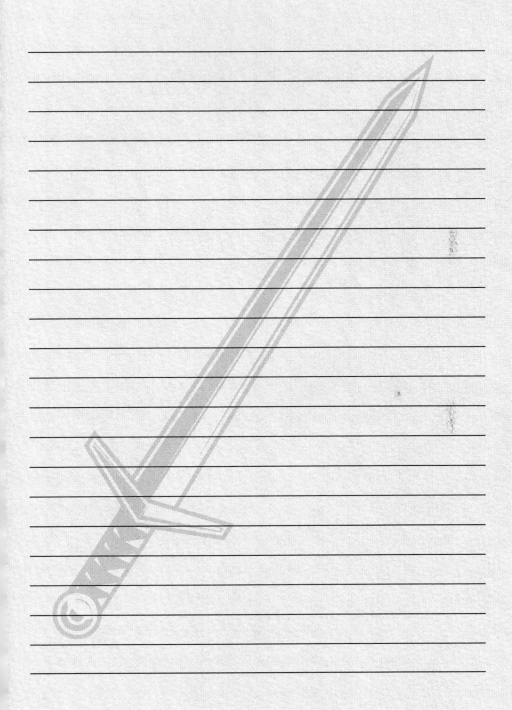

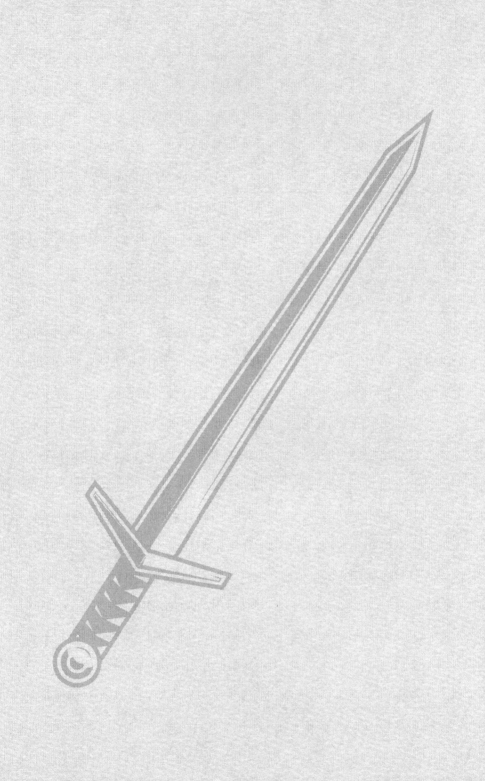

WEEKLY PLANNER
Week Four

MONDAY

TUESDAY

WEDNESDAY

THURSDAY

FRIDAY

SATURDAY

SUNDAY

BEDTIME FOR THE WEEK:

DID I GO TO CHURCH?
☐ Yes ☐ No

IF SO, WAS I LATE?
☐ Yes ☐ No

GOAL FOR THE FUTURE:

DAYS I WILL STUDY FOR IT:

WEEKLY POSITIVE QUOTE:

Be strong and courageous. Do not be afraid or terrified because of them, for the LORD your God goes with you; he will never leave you nor forsake you.

-Deuteronomy 31:6

Day 1

DID I?

Eat healthy?
Yes   No

Eat when I wasn't hungry?
Yes   No

Work out?
Yes   No
If yes, what did I do?
_____

Walk/Run one mile?
Yes   No

Read 15 pages/chapters?
Yes   No
If yes, what did I read?
_____

Pray 15 minutes?
Yes   No

Eat fruit/vegetables?
Yes   No

Listen to a Christian Podcast?
Yes   No
If yes, what did I listen to?
_____

Rest without napping?
Yes   No

Five things I did good or like about myself today:

1. _____
2. _____
3. _____
4. _____
5. _____

One thing I could do better: _____

How can I achieve it? _____

_____

NOTES

Day 2

DID I?

Eat healthy?
Yes   No

Eat when I wasn't hungry?
Yes   No

Work out?
Yes   No
If yes, what did I do?
_____

Walk/Run one mile?
Yes   No

Read 15 pages/chapters?
Yes   No
If yes, what did I read?
_____

Pray 15 minutes?
Yes   No

Eat fruit/vegetables?
Yes   No

Listen to a Christian Podcast?
Yes   No
If yes, what did I listen to?
_____

Rest without napping?
Yes   No

Five things I did good or like about myself today:

1._____
2._____
3._____
4._____
5._____

One thing I could do better: _____

How can I achieve it? _____

_____

NOTES

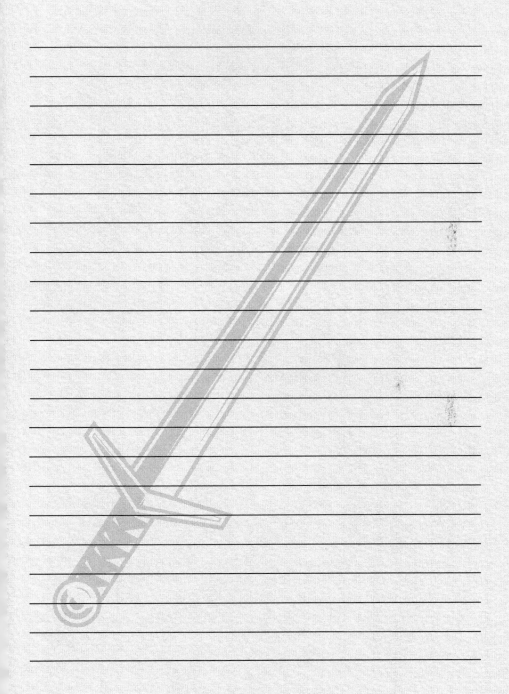

Day 3

DID I?

Eat healthy?
Yes   No

Eat when I wasn't hungry?
Yes   No

Work out?
Yes   No
If yes, what did I do?
_____

Walk/Run one mile?
Yes   No

Read 15 pages/chapters?
Yes   No
If yes, what did I read?
_____

Pray 15 minutes?
Yes   No

Eat fruit/vegetables?
Yes   No

Listen to a Christian Podcast?
Yes   No
If yes, what did I listen to?
_____

Rest without napping?
Yes   No

Five things I did good or like about myself today:

1._____
2._____
3._____
4._____
5._____

One thing I could do better: _____

How can I achieve it? _____
_____

NOTES

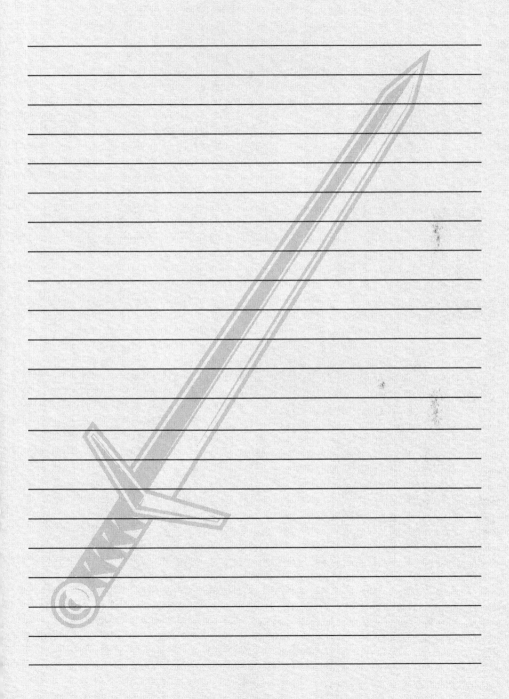

Day 4

DID I?

Eat healthy?
Yes   No

Eat when I
wasn't hungry?
Yes   No

Work out?
Yes   No
If yes, what did I do?
_____

Walk/Run one mile?
Yes   No

Read 15 pages/chapters?
Yes   No
If yes, what did I read?
_____

Pray 15 minutes?
Yes   No

Eat fruit/vegetables?
Yes   No

Listen to a Christian
Podcast?
Yes   No
If yes, what did I listen to?
_____

Rest without napping?
Yes   No

**Five things I did
good or like about
myself today:**

1._____
2._____
3._____
4._____
5._____

One thing I could do better: _____

How can I achieve it?   _____

_____

NOTES

Day 5

DID I?

Eat healthy?
Yes   No

Eat when I
wasn't hungry?
Yes   No

Work out?
Yes   No
If yes, what did I do?
_____

Walk/Run one mile?
Yes   No

Read 15 pages/chapters?
Yes   No
If yes, what did I read?
_____

Pray 15 minutes?
Yes   No

Eat fruit/vegetables?
Yes   No

Listen to a Christian
Podcast?
Yes   No
If yes, what did I listen to?
_____

Rest without napping?
Yes   No

**Five things I did
good or like about
myself today:**

1._____
2._____
3._____
4._____
5._____

One thing I could do better: _____

How can I achieve it? _____

_____

NOTES

Day 6

DID I?

Eat healthy?
Yes   No

Eat when I
wasn't hungry?
Yes   No

Work out?
Yes   No
If yes, what did I do?
_____

Walk/Run one mile?
Yes   No

Read 15 pages/chapters?
Yes   No
If yes, what did I read?
_____

Pray 15 minutes?
Yes   No

Eat fruit/vegetables?
Yes   No

Listen to a Christian
Podcast?
Yes   No
If yes, what did I listen to?
_____

Rest without napping?
Yes   No

Five things I did good or like about myself today:

1._____
2._____
3._____
4._____
5._____

One thing I could do better: _____

How can I achieve it?   _____

_____

NOTES

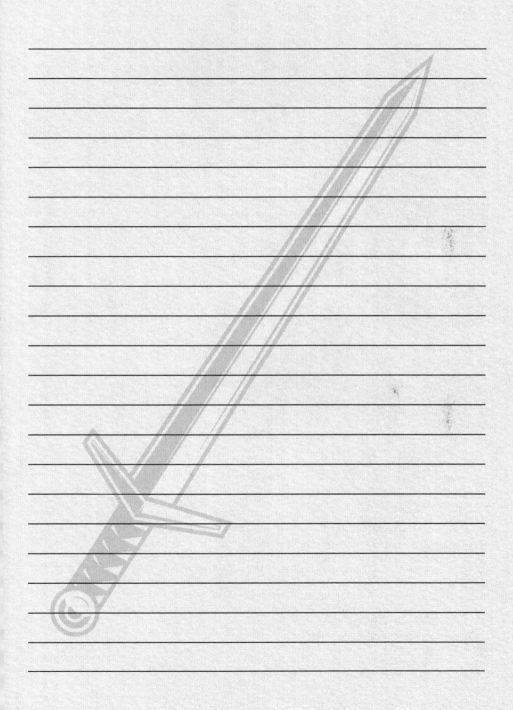

Day 7

DID I?

Eat healthy?
Yes   No

Eat when I wasn't hungry?
Yes   No

Work out?
Yes   No
If yes, what did I do?
_____

Walk/Run one mile?
Yes   No

Read 15 pages/chapters?
Yes   No
If yes, what did I read?
_____

Pray 15 minutes?
Yes   No

Eat fruit/vegetables?
Yes   No

Listen to a Christian Podcast?
Yes   No
If yes, what did I listen to?
_____

Rest without napping?
Yes   No

Five things I did good or like about myself today:

1. _____
2. _____
3. _____
4. _____
5. _____

One thing I could do better:

How can I achieve it?

_____
_____

NOTES

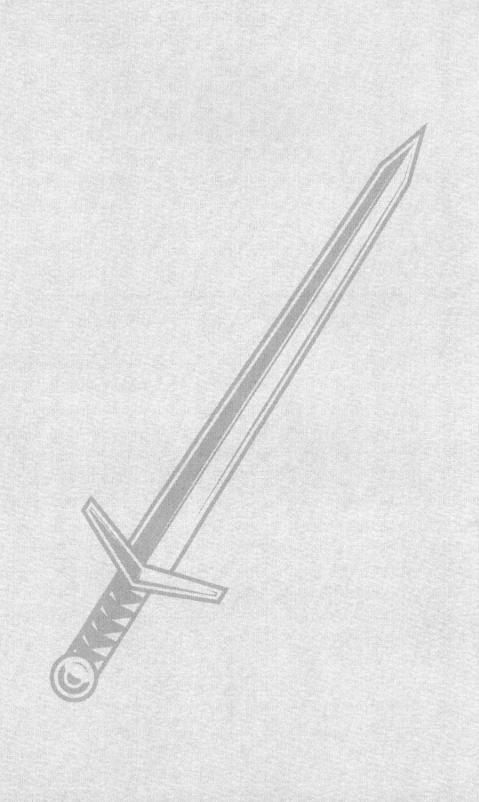

WEEKLY PLANNER

Week Five

MONDAY

TUESDAY

WEDNESDAY

THURSDAY

FRIDAY

SATURDAY

SUNDAY

BEDTIME FOR THE WEEK:

DID I GO TO CHURCH?
☐ Yes   ☐ No

IF SO, WAS I LATE?
☐ Yes   ☐ No

GOAL FOR THE FUTURE:

DAYS I WILL STUDY FOR IT:

WEEKLY POSITIVE QUOTE:

The steadfast love of the Lord never ceases; his mercies never come to an end; they are new every morning; great is your faithfulness.
                              -Lamentations 3:22-23

Day 1

DID I?

Eat healthy?
Yes   No

Eat when I wasn't hungry?
Yes   No

Work out?
Yes   No
If yes, what did I do?
_____

Walk/Run one mile?
Yes   No

Read 15 pages/chapters?
Yes   No
If yes, what did I read?
_____

Pray 15 minutes?
Yes   No

Eat fruit/vegetables?
Yes   No

Listen to a Christian Podcast?
Yes   No
If yes, what did I listen to?
_____

Rest without napping?
Yes   No

Five things I did good or like about myself today:

1._____
2._____
3._____
4._____
5._____

One thing I could do better: _____

How can I achieve it? _____

_____

NOTES

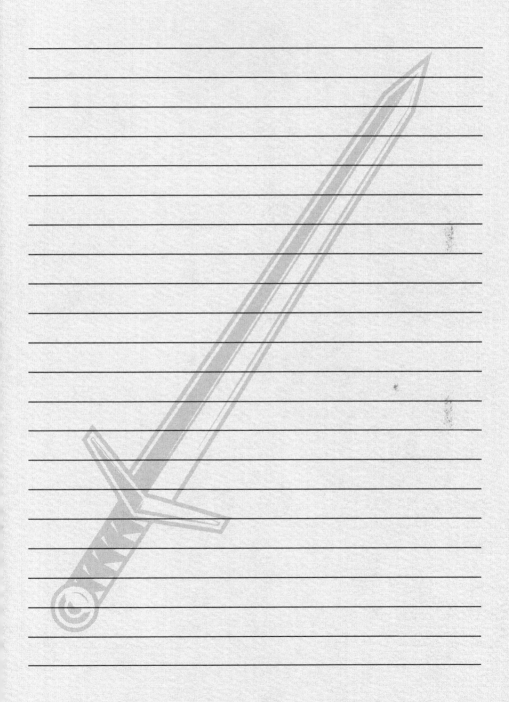

Day 2

DID I?

Eat healthy?
Yes   No

Eat when I
wasn't hungry?
Yes   No

Work out?
Yes   No
If yes, what did I do?
_____

Walk/Run one mile?
Yes   No

Read 15 pages/chapters?
Yes   No
If yes, what did I read?
_____

Pray 15 minutes?
Yes   No

Eat fruit/vegetables?
Yes   No

Listen to a Christian
Podcast?
Yes   No
If yes, what did I listen to?
_____

Rest without napping?
Yes   No

**Five things I did
good or like about
myself today:**

1._____
2._____
3._____
4._____
5._____

One thing I could do better: _____

How can I achieve it?   _____

_____

NOTES

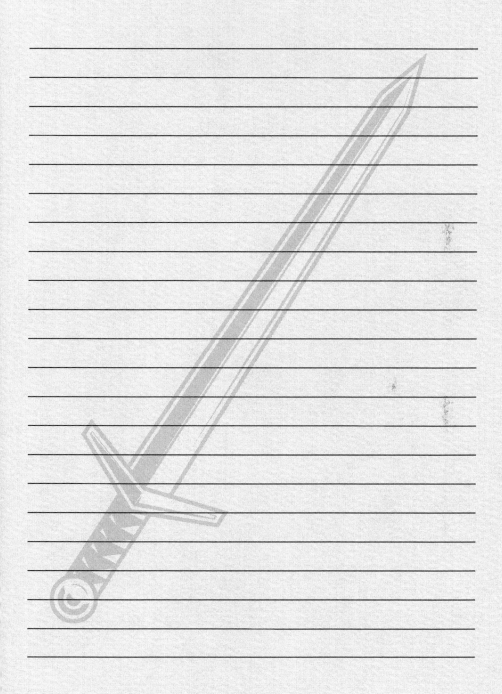

Day 3

DID I?

Eat healthy?
Yes   No

Eat when I wasn't hungry?
Yes   No

Work out?
Yes   No
If yes, what did I do?
_____

Walk/Run one mile?
Yes   No

Read 15 pages/chapters?
Yes   No
If yes, what did I read?
_____

Pray 15 minutes?
Yes   No

Eat fruit/vegetables?
Yes   No

Listen to a Christian Podcast?
Yes   No
If yes, what did I listen to?
_____

Rest without napping?
Yes   No

Five things I did good or like about myself today:

1._____
2._____
3._____
4._____
5._____

One thing I could do better: _____

How can I achieve it? _____
_____

NOTES

Day 4

DID I?

Eat healthy?
Yes   No

Eat when I
wasn't hungry?
Yes   No

Work out?
Yes   No
If yes, what did I do?
_____

Walk/Run one mile?
Yes   No

Read 15 pages/chapters?
Yes   No
If yes, what did I read?

_____

Pray 15 minutes?
Yes   No

Eat fruit/vegetables?
Yes   No

Listen to a Christian
Podcast?
Yes   No
If yes, what did I listen to?
_____

Rest without napping?
Yes   No

Five things I did
good or like about
myself today:

1._____
2._____
3._____
4._____
5._____

One thing I could do better: _____

How can I achieve it?   _____

_____

NOTES

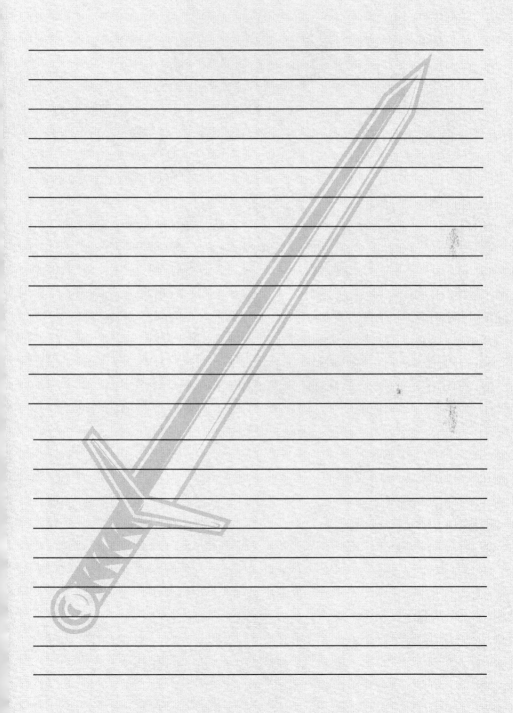

Day 5

DID I?

Eat healthy?
Yes   No

Eat when I wasn't hungry?
Yes   No

Work out?
Yes   No
If yes, what did I do?
_____

Walk/Run one mile?
Yes   No

Read 15 pages/chapters?
Yes   No
If yes, what did I read?
_____

Pray 15 minutes?
Yes   No

Eat fruit/vegetables?
Yes   No

Listen to a Christian Podcast?
Yes   No
If yes, what did I listen to?
_____

Rest without napping?
Yes   No

Five things I did good or like about myself today:

1._____
2._____
3._____
4._____
5._____

One thing I could do better: _____

How can I achieve it? _____
_____
_____

NOTES

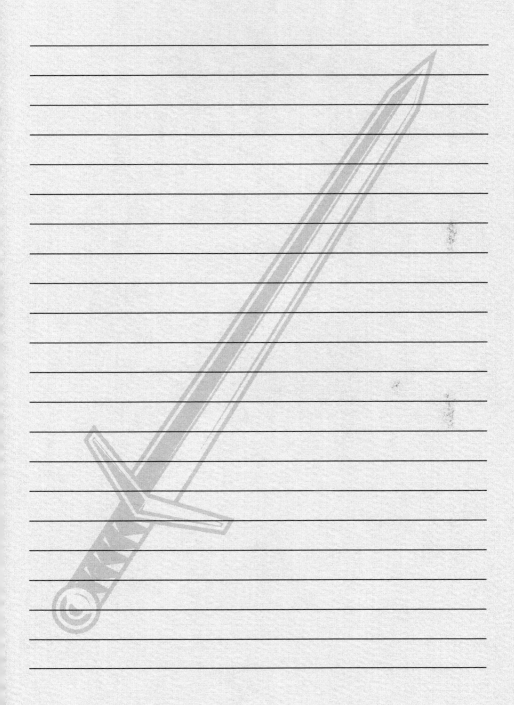

Day 6

DID I?

Eat healthy?
Yes   No

Eat when I wasn't hungry?
Yes   No

Work out?
Yes   No
If yes, what did I do?
_____

Walk/Run one mile?
Yes   No

Read 15 pages/chapters?
Yes   No
If yes, what did I read?
_____

Pray 15 minutes?
Yes   No

Eat fruit/vegetables?
Yes   No

Listen to a Christian Podcast?
Yes   No
If yes, what did I listen to?
_____

Rest without napping?
Yes   No

Five things I did good or like about myself today:

1. _____
2. _____
3. _____
4. _____
5. _____

One thing I could do better: _____

How can I achieve it? _____

_____

NOTES

Day 7

DID I?

Eat healthy?
Yes   No

Eat when I
wasn't hungry?
Yes   No

Work out?
Yes   No
If yes, what did I do?
_____

Walk/Run one mile?
Yes   No

Read 15 pages/chapters?
Yes   No
If yes, what did I read?
_____

Pray 15 minutes?
Yes   No

Eat fruit/vegetables?
Yes   No

Listen to a Christian
Podcast?
Yes   No
If yes, what did I listen to?
_____

Rest without napping?
Yes   No

Five things I did good or like about myself today:

1. _____
2. _____
3. _____
4. _____
5. _____

One thing I could do better: _____

How can I achieve it? _____
_____

NOTES

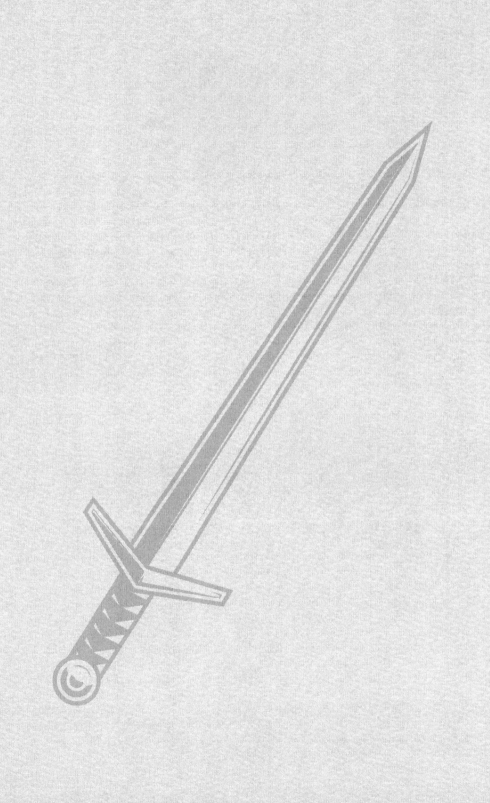

WEEKLY PLANNER

Week Six

MONDAY

TUESDAY

WEDNESDAY

THURSDAY

FRIDAY

SATURDAY

SUNDAY

BEDTIME FOR THE WEEK:

DID I GO TO CHURCH?
Yes   No

IF SO, WAS I LATE?
Yes   No

GOAL FOR THE FUTURE:

DAYS I WILL STUDY FOR IT:

WEEKLY POSITIVE QUOTE:

But those who hope in the LORD will renew their strength. They will soar on wings like eagles; they will run and not grow weary, they will walk and not be faint.

-Isaiah 40:31

Day 1

DID I?

Eat healthy?
Yes   No

Eat when I
wasn't hungry?
Yes   No

Work out?
Yes   No
If yes, what did I do?
_____

Walk/Run one mile?
Yes   No

Read 15 pages/chapters?
Yes   No
If yes, what did I read?
_____

Pray 15 minutes?
Yes   No

Eat fruit/vegetables?
Yes   No

Listen to a Christian
Podcast?
Yes   No
If yes, what did I listen to?
_____

Rest without napping?
Yes   No

**Five things I did
good or like about
myself today:**

1. _____
2. _____
3. _____
4. _____
5. _____

One thing I could do better: _____

How can I achieve it?   _____

_____

NOTES

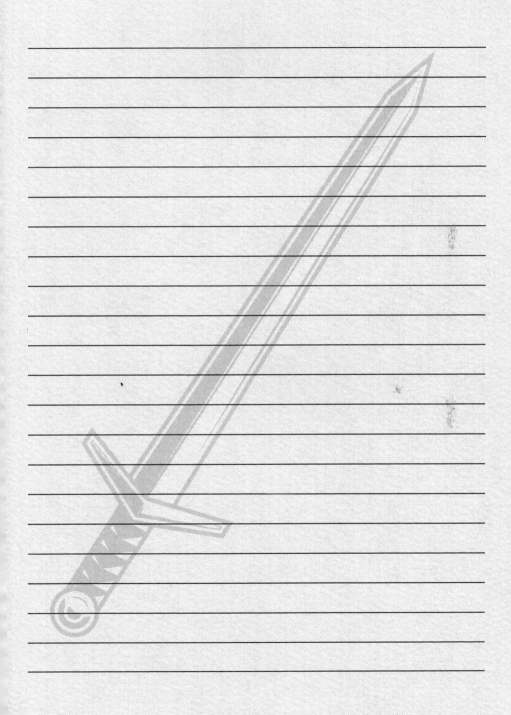

Day 2

DID I?

Eat healthy?
Yes   No

Eat when I wasn't hungry?
Yes   No

Work out?
Yes   No
If yes, what did I do?
_____

Walk/Run one mile?
Yes   No

Read 15 pages/chapters?
Yes   No
If yes, what did I read?
_____

Pray 15 minutes?
Yes   No

Eat fruit/vegetables?
Yes   No

Listen to a Christian Podcast?
Yes   No
If yes, what did I listen to?
_____

Rest without napping?
Yes   No

Five things I did good or like about myself today:

1._____
2._____
3._____
4._____
5._____

One thing I could do better: _____

How can I achieve it?   _____

_____

NOTES

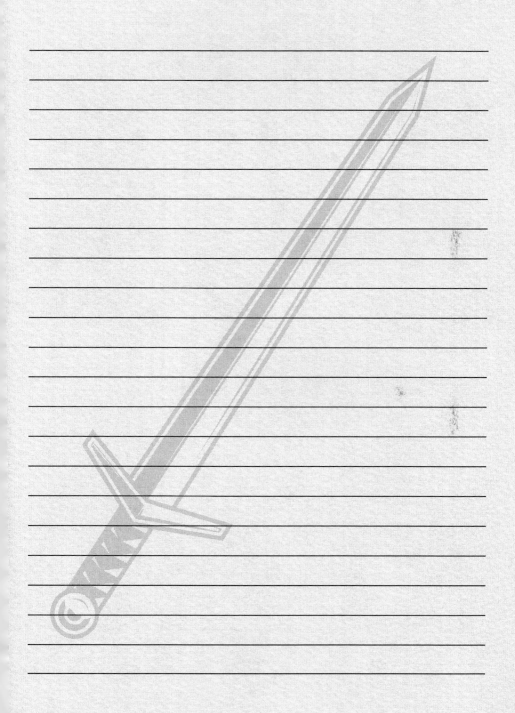

Day 3

DID I?

Eat healthy?
Yes   No

Eat when I
wasn't hungry?
Yes   No

Work out?
Yes   No
If yes, what did I do?
_____

Walk/Run one mile?
Yes   No

Read 15 pages/chapters?
Yes   No
If yes, what did I read?
_____

Pray 15 minutes?
Yes   No

Eat fruit/vegetables?
Yes   No

Listen to a Christian
Podcast?
Yes   No
If yes, what did I listen to?
_____

Rest without napping?
Yes   No

Five things I did good or like about myself today:

1. _____
2. _____
3. _____
4. _____
5. _____

One thing I could do better: _____

How can I achieve it? _____
_____

NOTES

Day 4

DID I?

Eat healthy?
Yes   No

Eat when I wasn't hungry?
Yes   No

Work out?
Yes   No
If yes, what did I do?
_____

Walk/Run one mile?
Yes   No

Read 15 pages/chapters?
Yes   No
If yes, what did I read?
_____

Pray 15 minutes?
Yes   No

Eat fruit/vegetables?
Yes   No

Listen to a Christian Podcast?
Yes   No
If yes, what did I listen to?
_____

Rest without napping?
Yes   No

Five things I did good or like about myself today:

1. _____
2. _____
3. _____
4. _____
5. _____

One thing I could do better: _____

How can I achieve it? _____
_____

NOTES

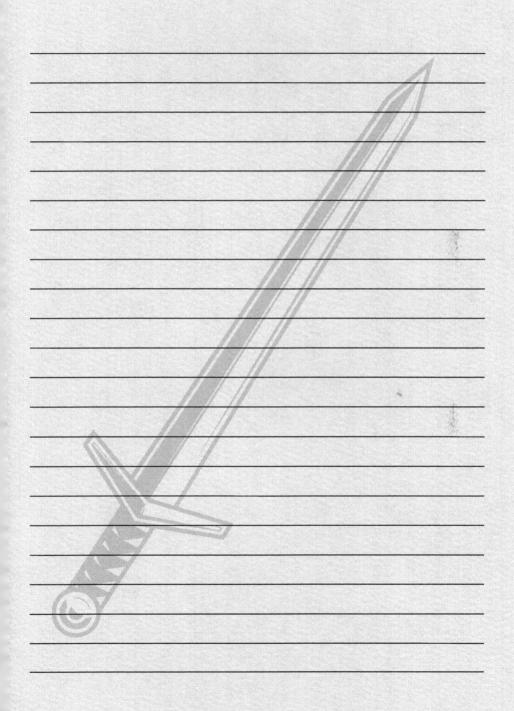

Day 5

DID I?

Eat healthy?
Yes   No

Eat when I wasn't hungry?
Yes   No

Work out?
Yes   No
If yes, what did I do?
_____

Walk/Run one mile?
Yes   No

Read 15 pages/chapters?
Yes   No
If yes, what did I read?
_____

Pray 15 minutes?
Yes   No

Eat fruit/vegetables?
Yes   No

Listen to a Christian Podcast?
Yes   No
If yes, what did I listen to?
_____

Rest without napping?
Yes   No

Five things I did good or like about myself today:

1._____
2._____
3._____
4._____
5._____

One thing I could do better: _____

How can I achieve it? _____
_____
_____

NOTES

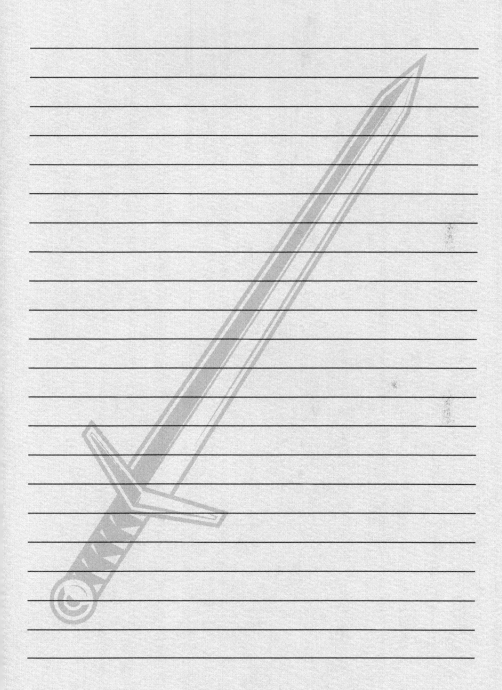

Day 6

DID I?

Eat healthy?
Yes   No

Eat when I
wasn't hungry?
Yes   No

Work out?
Yes   No
If yes, what did I do?
_____

Walk/Run one mile?
Yes   No

Read 15 pages/chapters?
Yes   No
If yes, what did I read?
_____

Pray 15 minutes?
Yes   No

Eat fruit/vegetables?
Yes   No

Listen to a Christian
Podcast?
Yes   No
If yes, what did I listen to?
_____

Rest without napping?
Yes   No

**Five things I did
good or like about
myself today:**

1. _____
2. _____
3. _____
4. _____
5. _____

One thing I could do better: _____

How can I achieve it?   _____

_____

NOTES

Day 7

DID I?

Eat healthy?
Yes   No

Eat when I wasn't hungry?
Yes   No

Work out?
Yes   No
If yes, what did I do?
_____

Walk/Run one mile?
Yes   No

Read 15 pages/chapters?
Yes   No
If yes, what did I read?
_____

Pray 15 minutes?
Yes   No

Eat fruit/vegetables?
Yes   No

Listen to a Christian Podcast?
Yes   No
If yes, what did I listen to?
_____

Rest without napping?
Yes   No

Five things I did good or like about myself today:

1. _____
2. _____
3. _____
4. _____
5. _____

One thing I could do better: _____

How can I achieve it? _____

_____

NOTES

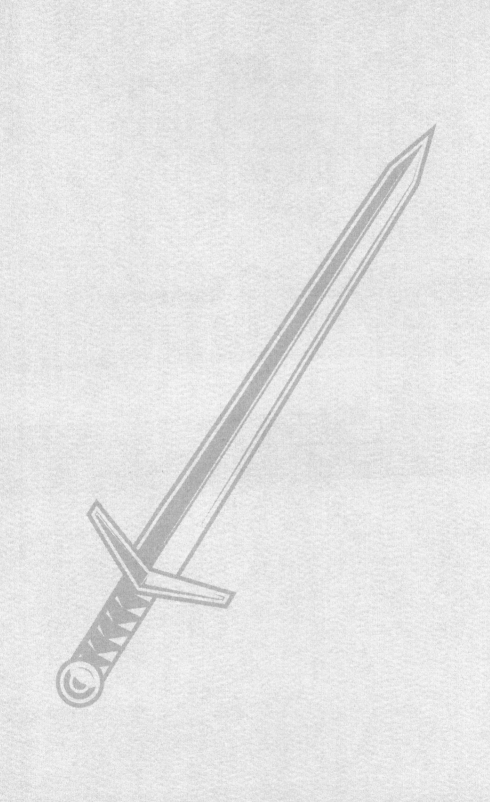

WEEKLY PLANNER
Week Seven

MONDAY

TUESDAY

WEDNESDAY

THURSDAY

FRIDAY

SATURDAY

SUNDAY

BEDTIME FOR THE WEEK:

DID I GO TO CHURCH?
☐ Yes ☐ No

IF SO, WAS I LATE?
☐ Yes ☐ No

GOAL FOR THE FUTURE:

DAYS I WILL STUDY FOR IT:

WEEKLY POSITIVE QUOTE:

Surely God is my salvation; I will trust and not be afraid. The LORD, the LORD himself, is my strength and my defense ; he has become my salvation.

~Isaiah 12:2

Day 1

DID I?

Eat healthy?
Yes   No

Eat when I wasn't hungry?
Yes   No

Work out?
Yes   No
If yes, what did I do?
_____

Walk/Run one mile?
Yes   No

Read 15 pages/chapters?
Yes   No
If yes, what did I read?
_____

Pray 15 minutes?
Yes   No

Eat fruit/vegetables?
Yes   No

Listen to a Christian Podcast?
Yes   No
If yes, what did I listen to?
_____

Rest without napping?
Yes   No

Five things I did good or like about myself today:

1._____
2._____
3._____
4._____
5._____

One thing I could do better: _____

How can I achieve it? _____
_____

NOTES

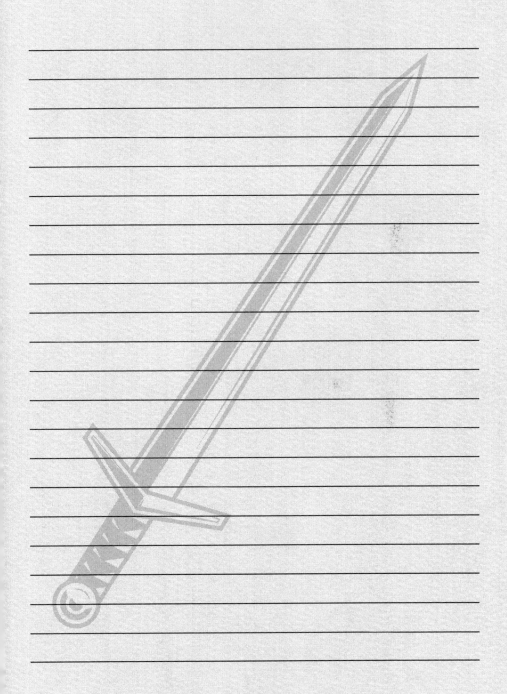

Day 2

DID I?

Eat healthy?
Yes   No

Eat when I wasn't hungry?
Yes   No

Work out?
Yes   No
If yes, what did I do?
_____

Walk/Run one mile?
Yes   No

Read 15 pages/chapters?
Yes   No
If yes, what did I read?
_____

Pray 15 minutes?
Yes   No

Eat fruit/vegetables?
Yes   No

Listen to a Christian Podcast?
Yes   No
If yes, what did I listen to?
_____

Rest without napping?
Yes   No

Five things I did good or like about myself today:

1. _____
2. _____
3. _____
4. _____
5. _____

One thing I could do better: _____

How can I achieve it? _____

_____

NOTES

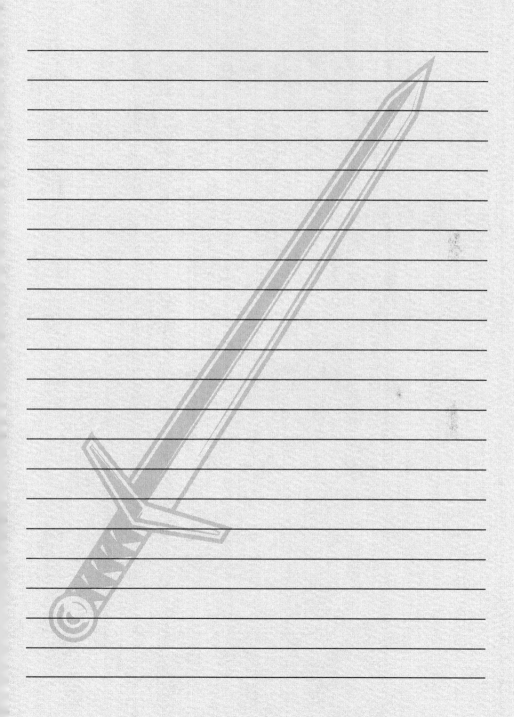

Day 3

DID I?

Eat healthy?
Yes   No

Eat when I wasn't hungry?
Yes   No

Work out?
Yes   No
If yes, what did I do?
_____

Walk/Run one mile?
Yes   No

Read 15 pages/chapters?
Yes   No
If yes, what did I read?
_____

Pray 15 minutes?
Yes   No

Eat fruit/vegetables?
Yes   No

Listen to a Christian Podcast?
Yes   No
If yes, what did I listen to?
_____

Rest without napping?
Yes   No

Five things I did good or like about myself today:

1._____
2._____
3._____
4._____
5._____

One thing I could do better: _____

How can I achieve it? _____
_____

NOTES

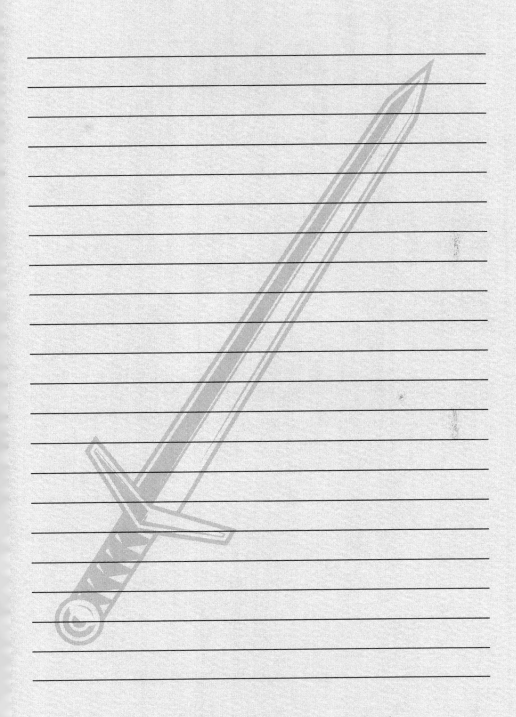

Day 4

DID I?

Eat healthy?
Yes   No

Eat when I
wasn't hungry?
Yes   No

Work out?
Yes   No
If yes, what did I do?
_____

Walk/Run one mile?
Yes   No

Read 15 pages/chapters?
Yes   No
If yes, what did I read?
_____

Pray 15 minutes?
Yes   No

Eat fruit/vegetables?
Yes   No

Listen to a Christian
Podcast?
Yes   No
If yes, what did I listen to?
_____

Rest without napping?
Yes   No

Five things I did good or like about myself today:

1._____
2._____
3._____
4._____
5._____

One thing I could do better: _____

How can I achieve it? _____

_____

NOTES

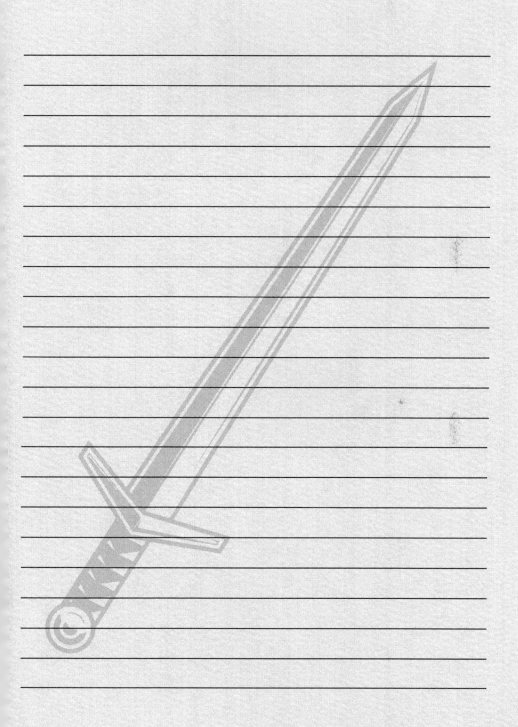

Day 5

DID I?

Eat healthy?
Yes   No

Eat when I wasn't hungry?
Yes   No

Work out?
Yes   No
If yes, what did I do?
_____

Walk/Run one mile?
Yes   No

Read 15 pages/chapters?
Yes   No
If yes, what did I read?
_____

Pray 15 minutes?
Yes   No

Eat fruit/vegetables?
Yes   No

Listen to a Christian Podcast?
Yes   No
If yes, what did I listen to?
_____

Rest without napping?
Yes   No

Five things I did good or like about myself today:

1. _____
2. _____
3. _____
4. _____
5. _____

One thing I could do better: _____

How can I achieve it? _____
_____

NOTES

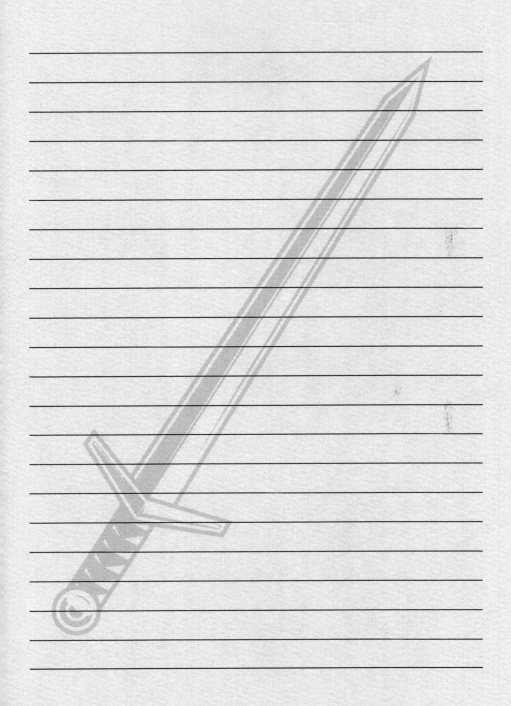

Day 6

DID I?

Eat healthy?
Yes   No

Eat when I wasn't hungry?
Yes   No

Work out?
Yes   No
If yes, what did I do?
_____

Walk/Run one mile?
Yes   No

Read 15 pages/chapters?
Yes   No
If yes, what did I read?
_____

Pray 15 minutes?
Yes   No

Eat fruit/vegetables?
Yes   No

Listen to a Christian Podcast?
Yes   No
If yes, what did I listen to?
_____

Rest without napping?
Yes   No

Five things I did good or like about myself today:

1. _____
2. _____
3. _____
4. _____
5. _____

One thing I could do better: _____

How can I achieve it? _____

_____

NOTES

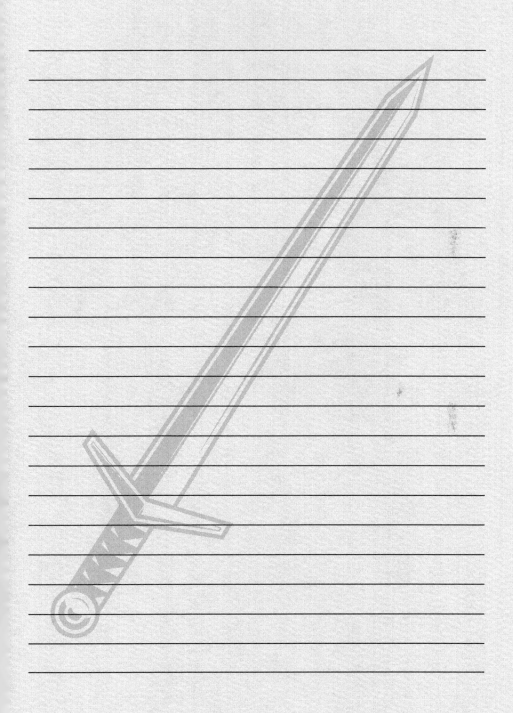

Day 7

DID I?

Eat healthy?
Yes   No

Eat when I
wasn't hungry?
Yes   No

Work out?
Yes   No
If yes, what did I do?

_____

Walk/Run one mile?
Yes   No

Read 15 pages/chapters?
Yes   No
If yes, what did I read?

_____

Pray 15 minutes?
Yes   No

Eat fruit/vegetables?
Yes   No

Rest without napping?
Yes   No

Listen to a Christian
Podcast?
Yes   No
If yes, what did I listen to?

_____

**Five things I did
good or like about
myself today:**

1. _____
2. _____
3. _____
4. _____
5. _____

One thing I could do better: _____

How can I achieve it? _____

NOTES

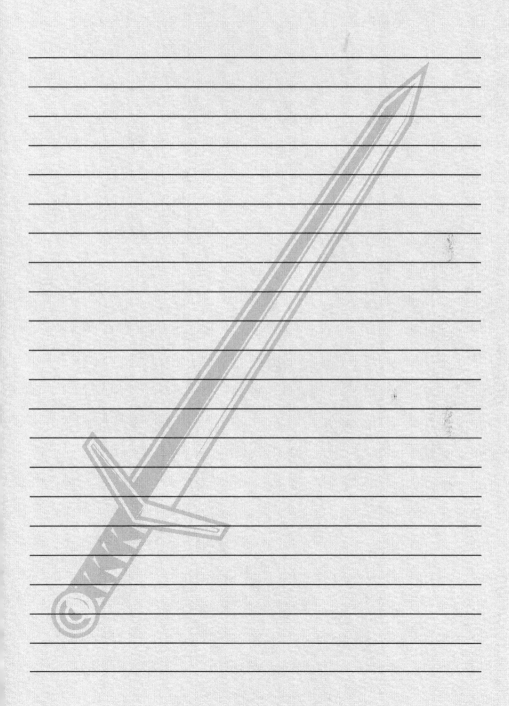

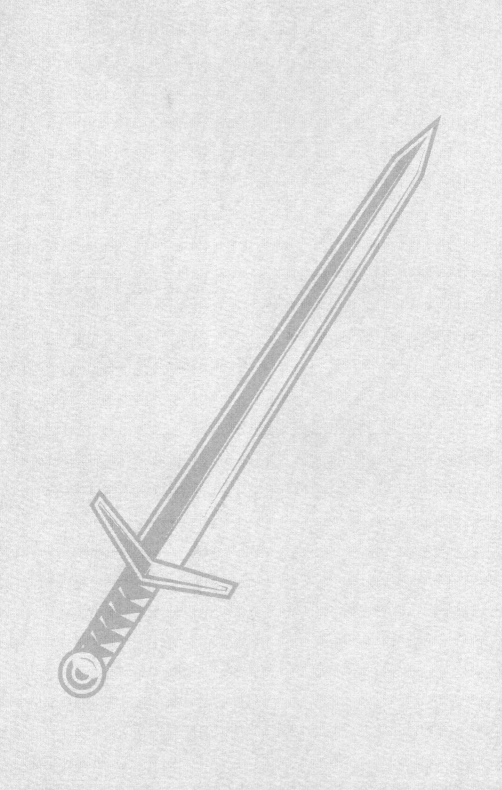

WEEKLY PLANNER
Week Eight

MONDAY

TUESDAY

WEDNESDAY

THURSDAY

FRIDAY

SATURDAY

SUNDAY

BEDTIME FOR THE WEEK:

DID I GO TO CHURCH?
☐ Yes   ☐ No

IF SO, WAS I LATE?
☐ Yes   ☐ No

GOAL FOR THE FUTURE:

DAYS I WILL STUDY FOR IT:

WEEKLY POSITIVE QUOTE:

When you pass through the waters, I will be with you; and when you pass through the rivers, they will not sweep over you. When you walk through the fire, you will not be burned; the flames will not set you ablaze.

~Isaiah 43:2

Day 1

DID I?

Eat healthy?
Yes   No

Eat when I
wasn't hungry?
Yes   No

Work out?
Yes   No
If yes, what did I do?
_____

Walk/Run one mile?
Yes   No

Read 15 pages/chapters?
Yes   No
If yes, what did I read?
_____

Pray 15 minutes?
Yes   No

Eat fruit/vegetables?
Yes   No

Listen to a Christian
Podcast?
Yes   No
If yes, what did I listen to?
_____

Rest without napping?
Yes   No

Five things I did good or like about myself today:

1. _____
2. _____
3. _____
4. _____
5. _____

One thing I could do better: _____

How can I achieve it?   _____

_____

NOTES

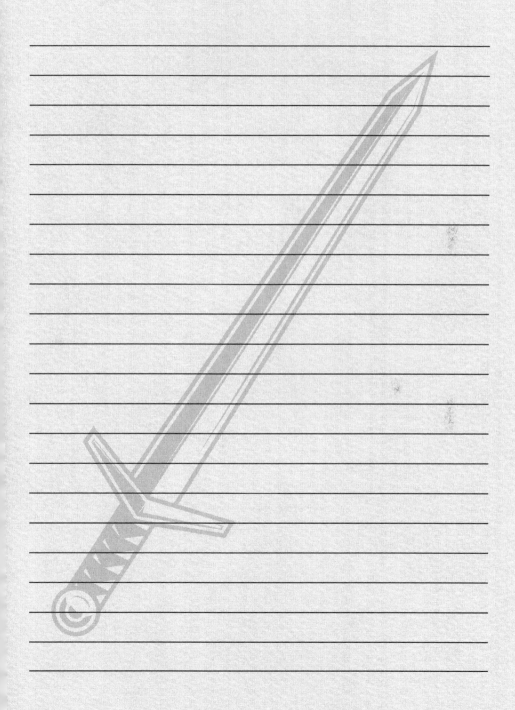

Day 2

DID I?

Eat healthy?
Yes   No

Eat when I wasn't hungry?
Yes   No

Work out?
Yes   No
If yes, what did I do?
_____

Walk/Run one mile?
Yes   No

Read 15 pages/chapters?
Yes   No
If yes, what did I read?
_____

Pray 15 minutes?
Yes   No

Eat fruit/vegetables?
Yes   No

Listen to a Christian Podcast?
Yes   No
If yes, what did I listen to?
_____

Rest without napping?
Yes   No

Five things I did good or like about myself today:

1. _____
2. _____
3. _____
4. _____
5. _____

One thing I could do better: _____

How can I achieve it? _____

_____

NOTES

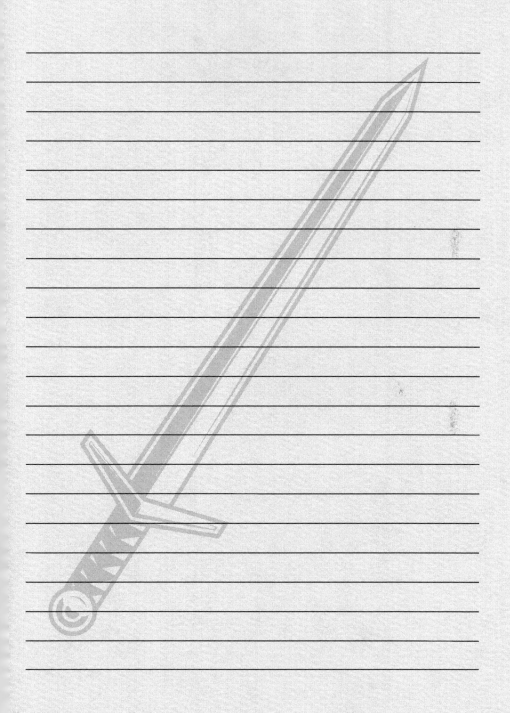

Day 3

DID I?

Eat healthy?
Yes   No

Eat when I wasn't hungry?
Yes   No

Work out?
Yes   No
If yes, what did I do?
_____

Walk/Run one mile?
Yes   No

Read 15 pages/chapters?
Yes   No
If yes, what did I read?
_____

Pray 15 minutes?
Yes   No

Eat fruit/vegetables?
Yes   No

Listen to a Christian Podcast?
Yes   No
If yes, what did I listen to?
_____

Rest without napping?
Yes   No

Five things I did good or like about myself today:

1. _____
2. _____
3. _____
4. _____
5. _____

One thing I could do better: _____

How can I achieve it? _____

_____

NOTES

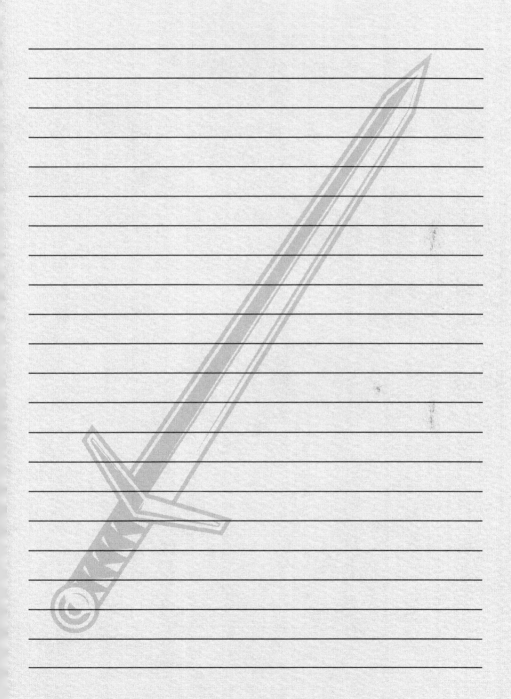

Day 4

DID I?

Eat healthy?
Yes   No

Eat when I
wasn't hungry?
Yes   No

Work out?
Yes   No
If yes, what did I do?
_____

Walk/Run one mile?
Yes   No

Read 15 pages/chapters?
Yes   No
If yes, what did I read?
_____

Pray 15 minutes?
Yes   No

Eat fruit/vegetables?
Yes   No

Listen to a Christian
Podcast?
Yes   No
If yes, what did I listen to?
_____

Rest without napping?
Yes   No

**Five things I did
good or like about
myself today:**

1._____
2._____
3._____
4._____
5._____

One thing I could do better: _____

How can I achieve it? _____

_____

NOTES

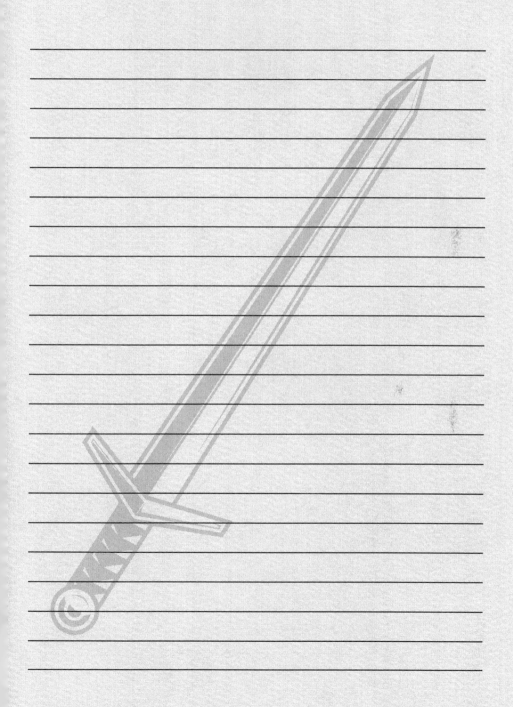

Day 5

DID I?

Eat healthy?
Yes   No

Eat when I wasn't hungry?
Yes   No

Work out?
Yes   No
If yes, what did I do?
_____

Walk/Run one mile?
Yes   No

Read 15 pages/chapters?
Yes   No
If yes, what did I read?
_____

Pray 15 minutes?
Yes   No

Eat fruit/vegetables?
Yes   No

Listen to a Christian Podcast?
Yes   No
If yes, what did I listen to?
_____

Rest without napping?
Yes   No

Five things I did good or like about myself today:

1._____
2._____
3._____
4._____
5._____

One thing I could do better: _____

How can I achieve it? _____
_____

NOTES

Day 6

DID I?

Eat healthy?
Yes   No

Eat when I
wasn't hungry?
Yes   No

Work out?
Yes   No
If yes, what did I do?
_____

Walk/Run one mile?
Yes   No

Read 15 pages/chapters?
Yes   No
If yes, what did I read?
_____

Pray 15 minutes?
Yes   No

Eat fruit/vegetables?
Yes   No

Listen to a Christian
Podcast?
Yes   No
If yes, what did I listen to?
_____

Rest without napping?
Yes   No

**Five things I did
good or like about
myself today:**

1. _____
2. _____
3. _____
4. _____
5. _____

One thing I could do better: _____

How can I achieve it?   _____

_____

NOTES

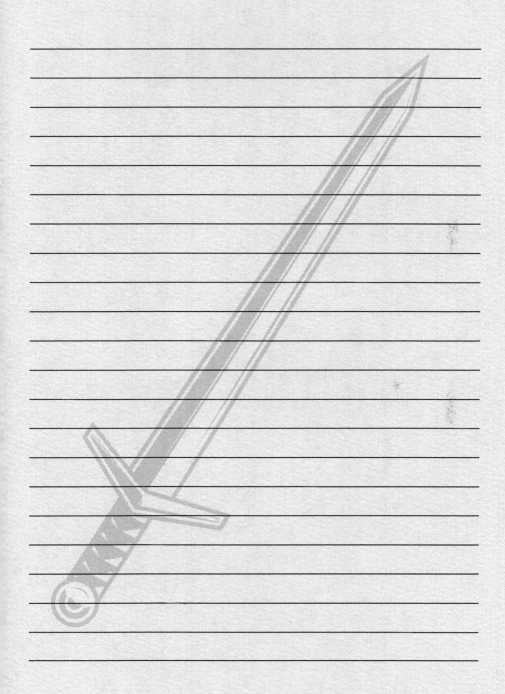

Day 7

DID I?

Eat healthy?
Yes   No

Eat when I wasn't hungry?
Yes   No

Work out?
Yes   No
If yes, what did I do?
_____

Walk/Run one mile?
Yes   No

Read 15 pages/chapters?
Yes   No
If yes, what did I read?
_____

Pray 15 minutes?
Yes   No

Eat fruit/vegetables?
Yes   No

Listen to a Christian Podcast?
Yes   No
If yes, what did I listen to?
_____

Rest without napping?
Yes   No

Five things I did good or like about myself today:

1. _____
2. _____
3. _____
4. _____
5. _____

One thing I could do better:

How can I achieve it?

_____
_____
_____

NOTES

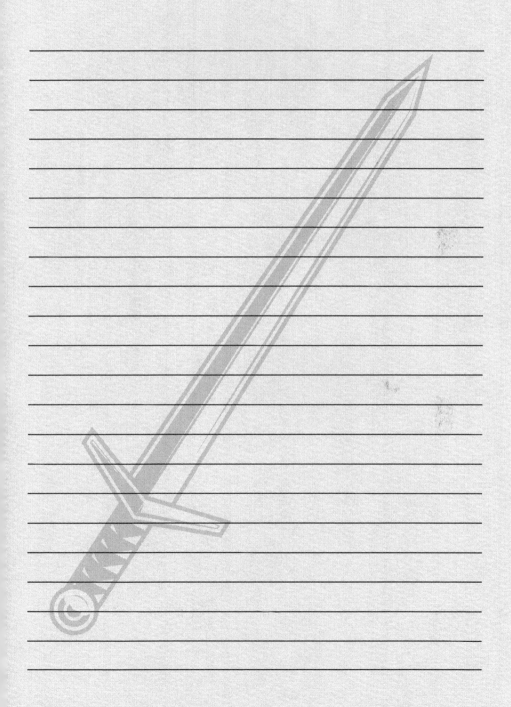

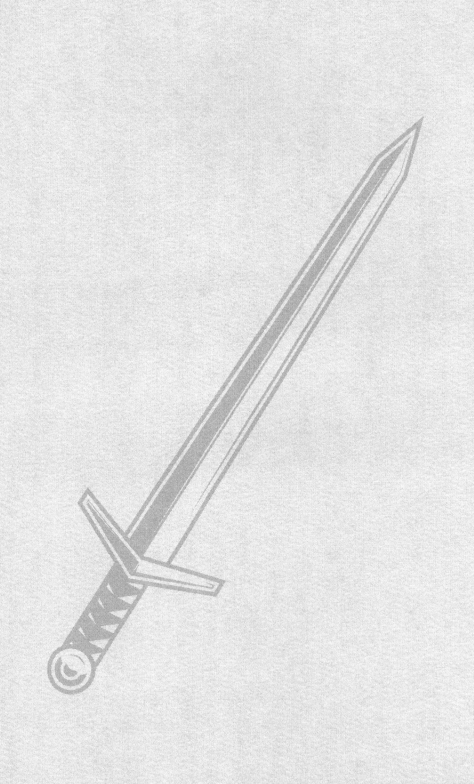

WEEKLY PLANNER

Week Nine

MONDAY

TUESDAY

WEDNESDAY

THURSDAY

FRIDAY

SATURDAY

SUNDAY

BEDTIME FOR THE WEEK:

DID I GO TO CHURCH?
☐ Yes ☐ No

IF SO, WAS I LATE?
☐ Yes ☐ No

GOAL FOR THE FUTURE:

DAYS I WILL STUDY FOR IT:

WEEKLY POSITIVE QUOTE:

The Lord your God is with you, the Mighty Warrior who saves. He will take great delight in you; in his love He will no longer rebuke you, but will rejoice over you with singing.
~Zephaniah 3:17 (NIV)

Day 1

DID I?

Eat healthy?
Yes   No

Eat when I wasn't hungry?
Yes   No

Work out?
Yes   No
If yes, what did I do?
_____

Walk/Run one mile?
Yes   No

Read 15 pages/chapters?
Yes   No
If yes, what did I read?
_____

Pray 15 minutes?
Yes   No

Eat fruit/vegetables?
Yes   No

Listen to a Christian Podcast?
Yes   No
If yes, what did I listen to?
_____

Rest without napping?
Yes   No

Five things I did good or like about myself today:

1. _____
2. _____
3. _____
4. _____
5. _____

One thing I could do better: _____

How can I achieve it? _____
_____
_____

NOTES

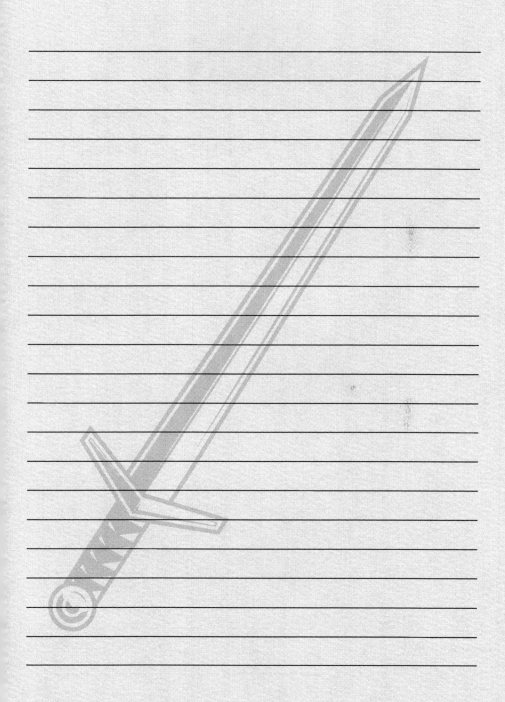

Day 2

DID I?

Eat healthy?
Yes   No

Eat when I wasn't hungry?
Yes   No

Work out?
Yes   No
If yes, what did I do?
_____

Walk/Run one mile?
Yes   No

Read 15 pages/chapters?
Yes   No
If yes, what did I read?
_____

Pray 15 minutes?
Yes   No

Eat fruit/vegetables?
Yes   No

Listen to a Christian Podcast?
Yes   No
If yes, what did I listen to?
_____

Rest without napping?
Yes   No

Five things I did good or like about myself today:

1._____
2._____
3._____
4._____
5._____

One thing I could do better: _____

How can I achieve it? _____

_____

NOTES

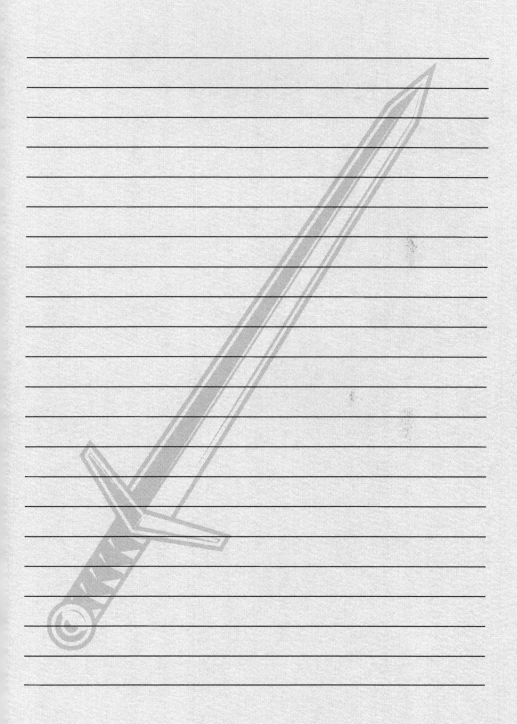

Day 3

DID I?

Eat healthy?
Yes   No

Eat when I wasn't hungry?
Yes   No

Work out?
Yes   No
If yes, what did I do?
_____

Walk/Run one mile?
Yes   No

Read 15 pages/chapters?
Yes   No
If yes, what did I read?
_____

Pray 15 minutes?
Yes   No

Eat fruit/vegetables?
Yes   No

Listen to a Christian Podcast?
Yes   No
If yes, what did I listen to?
_____

Rest without napping?
Yes   No

Five things I did good or like about myself today:

1._____
2._____
3._____
4._____
5._____

One thing I could do better: _____

How can I achieve it? _____

_____

NOTES

Day 4

DID I?

Eat healthy?
Yes   No

Eat when I wasn't hungry?
Yes   No

Work out?
Yes   No
If yes, what did I do?
_____

Walk/Run one mile?
Yes   No

Read 15 pages/chapters?
Yes   No
If yes, what did I read?
_____

Pray 15 minutes?
Yes   No

Eat fruit/vegetables?
Yes   No

Listen to a Christian Podcast?
Yes   No
If yes, what did I listen to?
_____

Rest without napping?
Yes   No

Five things I did good or like about myself today:

1._____
2._____
3._____
4._____
5._____

One thing I could do better: _____

How can I achieve it? _____

_____

NOTES

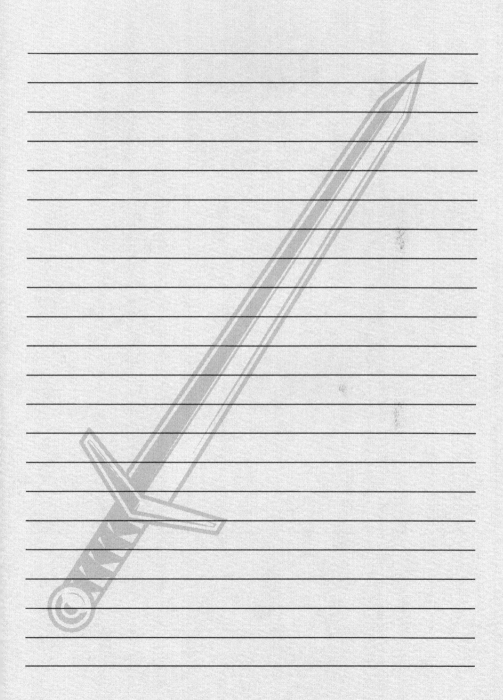

Day 5

DID I?

Eat healthy?
Yes   No

Eat when I wasn't hungry?
Yes   No

Work out?
Yes   No
If yes, what did I do?
_____

Walk/Run one mile?
Yes   No

Read 15 pages/chapters?
Yes   No
If yes, what did I read?
_____

Pray 15 minutes?
Yes   No

Eat fruit/vegetables?
Yes   No

Listen to a Christian Podcast?
Yes   No
If yes, what did I listen to?
_____

Rest without napping?
Yes   No

Five things I did good or like about myself today:

1. _____
2. _____
3. _____
4. _____
5. _____

One thing I could do better:

_____

How can I achieve it?

_____

_____

NOTES

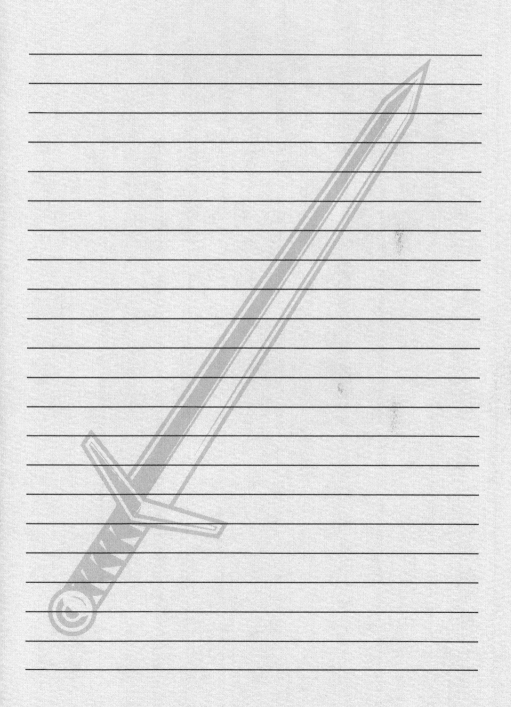

Day 6

DID I?

Eat healthy?
Yes   No

Eat when I
wasn't hungry?
Yes   No

Work out?
Yes   No
If yes, what did I do?
_____

Walk/Run one mile?
Yes   No

Read 15 pages/chapters?
Yes   No
If yes, what did I read?
_____

Pray 15 minutes?
Yes   No

Eat fruit/vegetables?
Yes   No

Listen to a Christian
Podcast?
Yes   No
If yes, what did I listen to?
_____

Rest without napping?
Yes   No

Five things I did good or like about myself today:

1. _____
2. _____
3. _____
4. _____
5. _____

One thing I could do better: _____

How can I achieve it?   _____

_____

NOTES

Day 7

DID I?

Eat healthy?
Yes   No

Eat when I wasn't hungry?
Yes   No

Work out?
Yes   No
If yes, what did I do?
_____

Walk/Run one mile?
Yes   No

Read 15 pages/chapters?
Yes   No
If yes, what did I read?
_____

Pray 15 minutes?
Yes   No

Eat fruit/vegetables?
Yes   No

Listen to a Christian Podcast?
Yes   No
If yes, what did I listen to?
_____

Rest without napping?
Yes   No

Five things I did good or like about myself today:

1. _____
2. _____
3. _____
4. _____
5. _____

One thing I could do better: _____

How can I achieve it? _____

NOTES

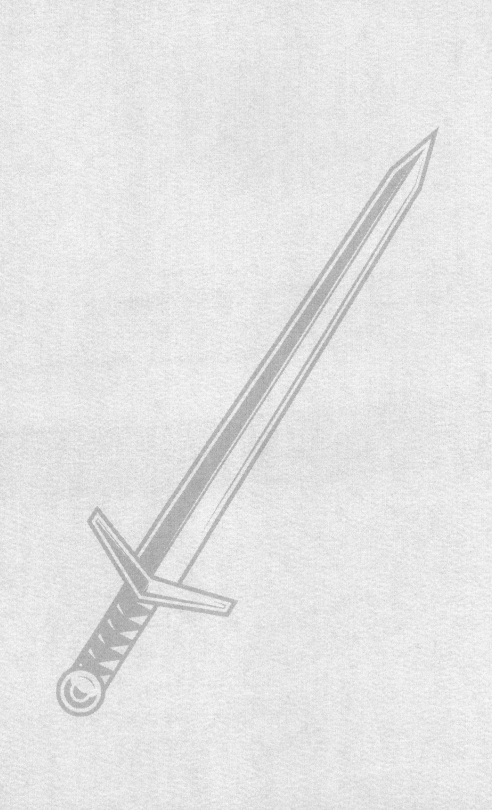

WEEKLY PLANNER
Week Ten

MONDAY

TUESDAY

WEDNESDAY

THURSDAY

FRIDAY

SATURDAY

SUNDAY

BEDTIME FOR THE WEEK:

DID I GO TO CHURCH?
☐ Yes   ☐ No

IF SO, WAS I LATE?
☐ Yes   ☐ No

GOAL FOR THE FUTURE:

DAYS I WILL STUDY FOR IT:

WEEKLY POSITIVE QUOTE:

Do not be anxious about anything, but in every situation, by prayer and petition, with thanksgiving, present your requests to God. And the peace of God, which transcends all understanding, will guard your hearts and your minds in Christ Jesus.

-Philippians 4:6–7 (NIV)

Day 1

DID I?

Eat healthy?
Yes   No

Eat when I wasn't hungry?
Yes   No

Work out?
Yes   No
If yes, what did I do?
_____

Walk/Run one mile?
Yes   No

Read 15 pages/chapters?
Yes   No
If yes, what did I read?
_____

Pray 15 minutes?
Yes   No

Eat fruit/vegetables?
Yes   No

Listen to a Christian Podcast?
Yes   No
If yes, what did I listen to?
_____

Rest without napping?
Yes   No

Five things I did good or like about myself today:

1._____
2._____
3._____
4._____
5._____

One thing I could do better: _____

How can I achieve it? _____
_____

NOTES

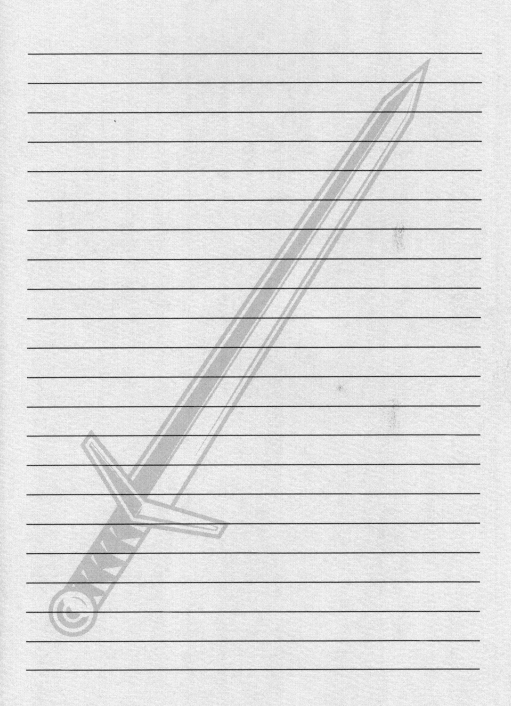

Day 2

DID I?

Eat healthy?
Yes   No

Eat when I wasn't hungry?
Yes   No

Work out?
Yes   No
If yes, what did I do?
_____

Walk/Run one mile?
Yes   No

Read 15 pages/chapters?
Yes   No
If yes, what did I read?
_____

Pray 15 minutes?
Yes   No

Eat fruit/vegetables?
Yes   No

Listen to a Christian Podcast?
Yes   No
If yes, what did I listen to?
_____

Rest without napping?
Yes   No

Five things I did good or like about myself today:

1._____
2._____
3._____
4._____
5._____

One thing I could do better: _____

How can I achieve it?   _____
_____

NOTES

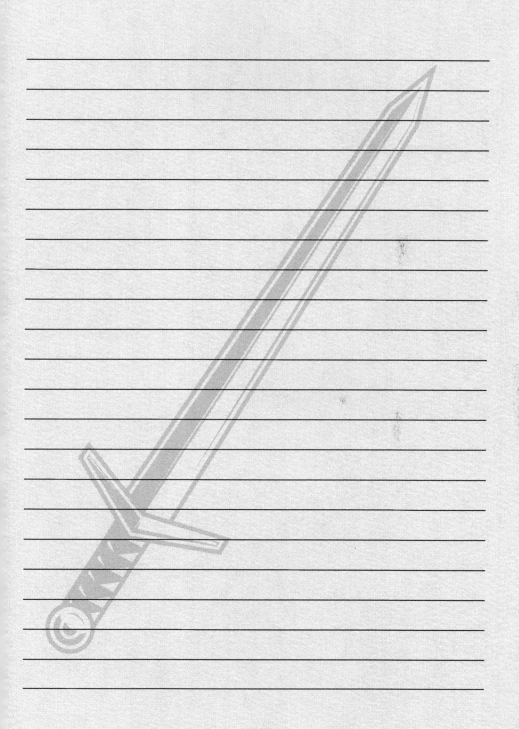

Day 3

DATE: / /

DID I?

Eat healthy?
Yes   No

Eat when I
wasn't hungry?
Yes   No

Work out?
Yes   No
If yes, what did I do?
_____

Walk/Run one mile?
Yes   No

Read 15 pages/chapters?
Yes   No
If yes, what did I read?
_____

Pray 15 minutes?
Yes   No

Eat fruit/vegetables?
Yes   No

Listen to a Christian
Podcast?
Yes   No
If yes, what did I listen to?
_____

Rest without napping?
Yes   No

Five things I did good or like about myself today:

1. _____
2. _____
3. _____
4. _____
5. _____

One thing I could do better: _____

How can I achieve it? _____

_____

NOTES

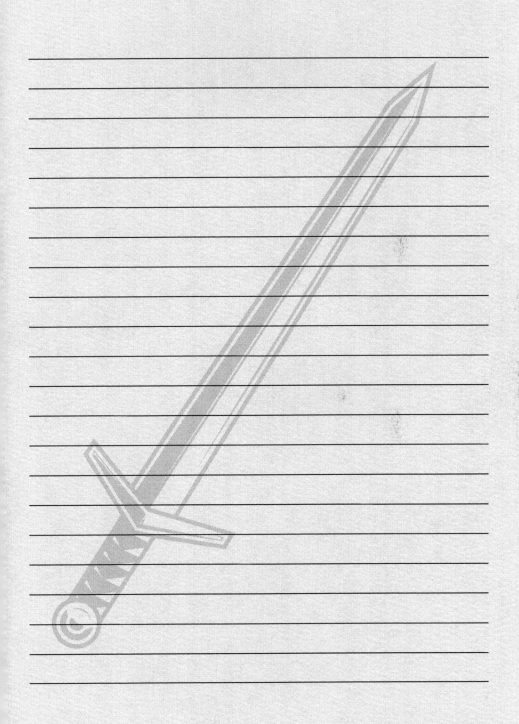

Day 4

DATE: / /

DID I?

Eat healthy?
Yes   No

Eat when I wasn't hungry?
Yes   No

Work out?
Yes   No
If yes, what did I do?
_____

Walk/Run one mile?
Yes   No

Read 15 pages/chapters?
Yes   No
If yes, what did I read?
_____

Pray 15 minutes?
Yes   No

Eat fruit/vegetables?
Yes   No

Listen to a Christian Podcast?
Yes   No
If yes, what did I listen to?
_____

Rest without napping?
Yes   No

Five things I did good or like about myself today:

1. _____
2. _____
3. _____
4. _____
5. _____

One thing I could do better: _____

How can I achieve it? _____
_____

NOTES

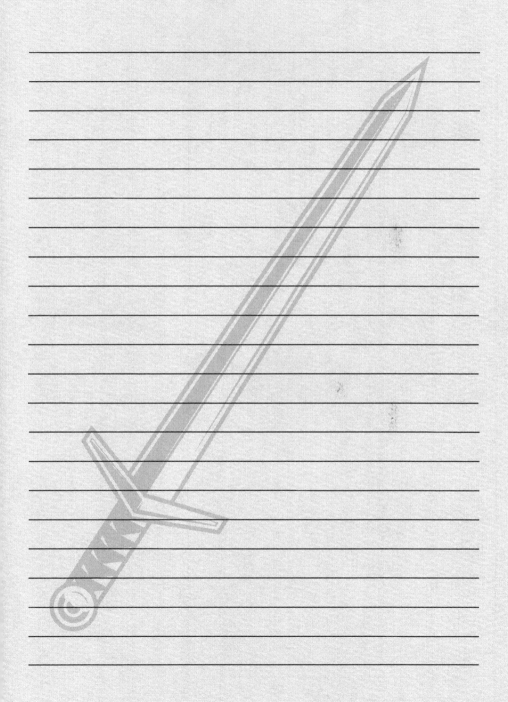

Day 5

DID I?

Eat healthy?
Yes   No

Eat when I
wasn't hungry?
Yes   No

Work out?
Yes   No
If yes, what did I do?
_____

Walk/Run one mile?
Yes   No

Read 15 pages/chapters?
Yes   No
If yes, what did I read?

_____

Pray 15 minutes?
Yes   No

Eat fruit/vegetables?
Yes   No

Listen to a Christian
Podcast?
Yes   No
If yes, what did I listen to?
_____

Rest without napping?
Yes   No

**Five things I did
good or like about
myself today:**

1._____
2._____
3._____
4._____
5._____

One thing I could do better: _____

How can I achieve it?   _____

_____

NOTES

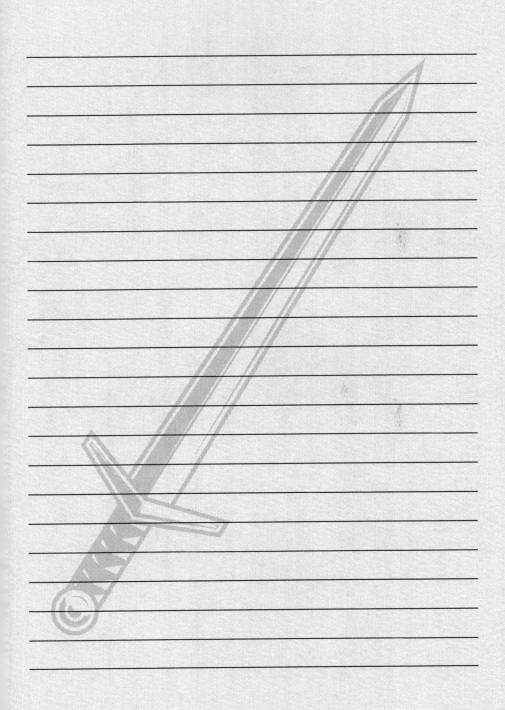

Day 6

DID I?

Eat healthy?
Yes   No

Eat when I wasn't hungry?
Yes   No

Work out?
Yes   No
If yes, what did I do?
_____

Walk/Run one mile?
Yes   No

Read 15 pages/chapters?
Yes   No
If yes, what did I read?
_____

Pray 15 minutes?
Yes   No

Eat fruit/vegetables?
Yes   No

Listen to a Christian Podcast?
Yes   No
If yes, what did I listen to?
_____

Rest without napping?
Yes   No

Five things I did good or like about myself today:

1. _____
2. _____
3. _____
4. _____
5. _____

One thing I could do better: _____

How can I achieve it? _____

_____

NOTES

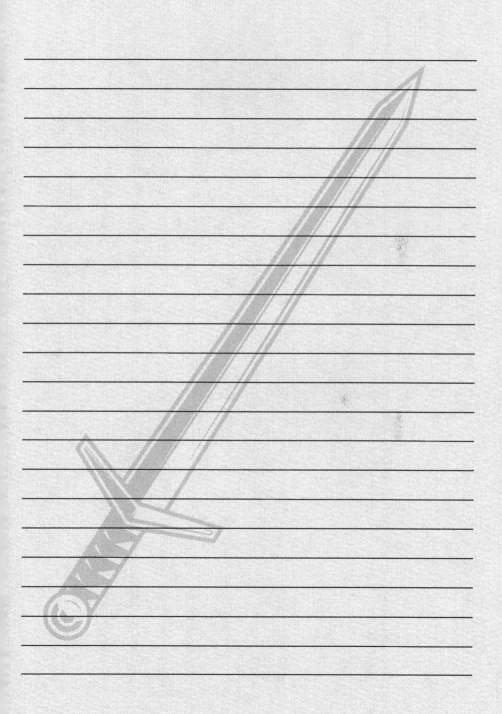

Day 7

DID I?

Eat healthy?
Yes   No

Eat when I wasn't hungry?
Yes   No

Work out?
Yes   No
If yes, what did I do?
_____

Walk/Run one mile?
Yes   No

Read 15 pages/chapters?
Yes   No
If yes, what did I read?
_____

Pray 15 minutes?
Yes   No

Eat fruit/vegetables?
Yes   No

Listen to a Christian Podcast?
Yes   No
If yes, what did I listen to?
_____

Rest without napping?
Yes   No

Five things I did good or like about myself today:

1. _____
2. _____
3. _____
4. _____
5. _____

One thing I could do better:

How can I achieve it?
_____
_____

NOTES

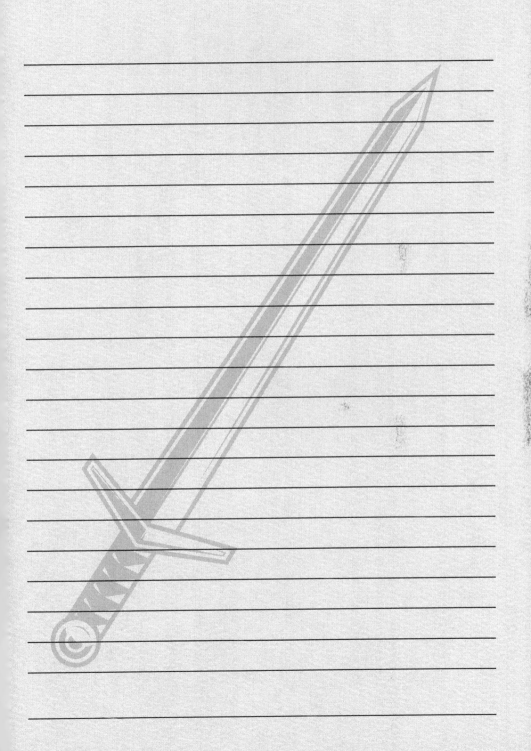

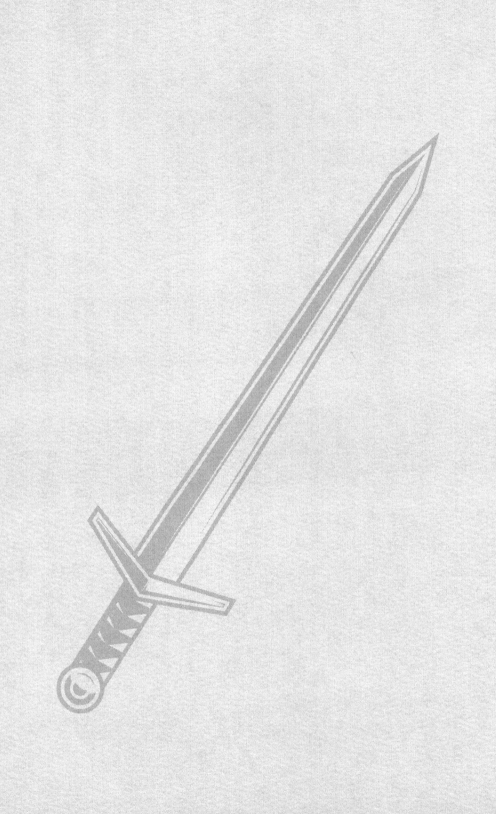

WEEKLY PLANNER

Week Eleven

MONDAY

TUESDAY

WEDNESDAY

THURSDAY

FRIDAY

SATURDAY

SUNDAY

BEDTIME FOR THE WEEK:

DID I GO TO CHURCH?
☐ Yes ☐ No

IF SO, WAS I LATE?
☐ Yes ☐ No

GOAL FOR THE FUTURE:

DAYS I WILL STUDY FOR IT:

WEEKLY POSITIVE QUOTE:

Therefore we do not lose heart. Though outwardly we are wasting away, yet inwardly we are being renewed day by day. For our light and momentary troubles are achieving for us an eternal glory that far outweighs them all. So we fix our eyes not on what is seen, but on what is unseen, since what is seen is temporary, but what is unseen is eternal.

~2 Corinthians 4:16-18 (NIV)

Day 1

DATE: /   /

DID I?

Eat healthy?
Yes   No

Eat when I wasn't hungry?
Yes   No

Work out?
Yes   No
If yes, what did I do?
_____

Walk/Run one mile?
Yes   No

Read 15 pages/chapters?
Yes   No
If yes, what did I read?

_____

Pray 15 minutes?
Yes   No

Eat fruit/vegetables?
Yes   No

Listen to a Christian Podcast?
Yes   No
If yes, what did I listen to?
_____

Rest without napping?
Yes   No

Five things I did good or like about myself today:

1. _____
2. _____
3. _____
4. _____
5. _____

One thing I could do better: _____

How can I achieve it? _____

_____

NOTES

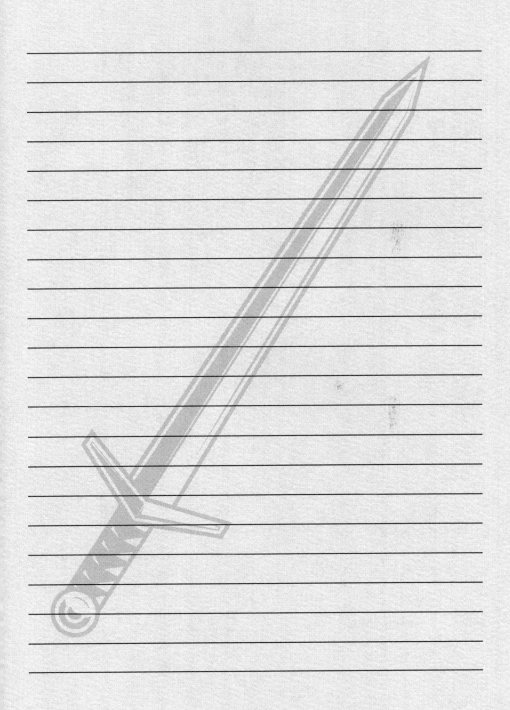

Day 2

DATE: / /

DID I?

Eat healthy?
Yes   No

Eat when I
wasn't hungry?
Yes   No

Work out?
Yes   No
If yes, what did I do?
_____

Walk/Run one mile?
Yes   No

Read 15 pages/chapters?
Yes   No
If yes, what did I read?
_____

Pray 15 minutes?
Yes   No

Eat fruit/vegetables?
Yes   No

Listen to a Christian
Podcast?
Yes   No
If yes, what did I listen to?
_____

Rest without napping?
Yes   No

Five things I did good or like about myself today:

1. _____
2. _____
3. _____
4. _____
5. _____

One thing I could do better: _____

How can I achieve it? _____

_____

NOTES

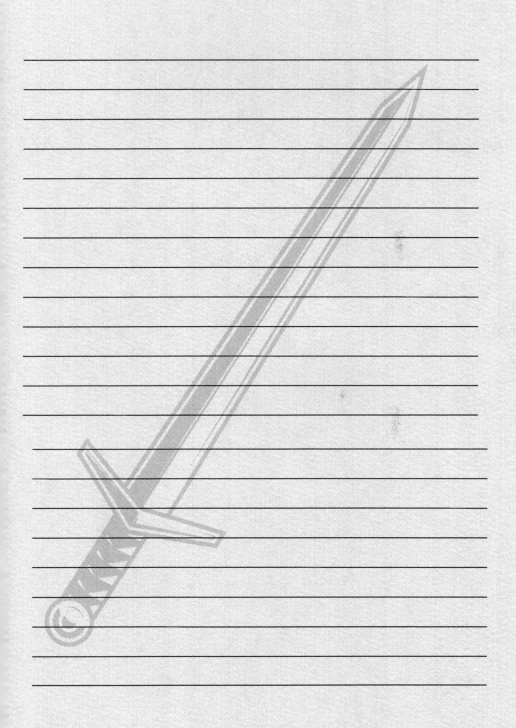

Day 3

DID I?

Eat healthy?
Yes   No

Eat when I
wasn't hungry?
Yes   No

Work out?
Yes   No
If yes, what did I do?
_____

Walk/Run one mile?
Yes   No

Read 15 pages/chapters?
Yes   No
If yes, what did I read?
_____

Pray 15 minutes?
Yes   No

Eat fruit/vegetables?
Yes   No

Listen to a Christian
Podcast?
Yes   No
If yes, what did I listen to?
_____

Rest without napping?
Yes   No

Five things I did good or like about myself today:

1. _____
2. _____
3. _____
4. _____
5. _____

One thing I could do better: _____

How can I achieve it? _____

_____

NOTES

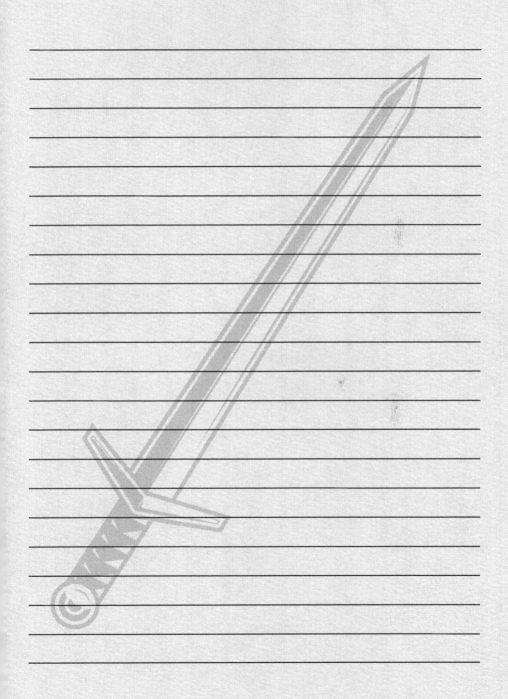

Day 4

DID I?

Eat healthy?
Yes   No

Eat when I wasn't hungry?
Yes   No

Work out?
Yes   No
If yes, what did I do?
_____

Walk/Run one mile?
Yes   No

Read 15 pages/chapters?
Yes   No
If yes, what did I read?
_____

Pray 15 minutes?
Yes   No

Eat fruit/vegetables?
Yes   No

Listen to a Christian Podcast?
Yes   No
If yes, what did I listen to?
_____

Rest without napping?
Yes   No

Five things I did good or like about myself today:

1._____
2._____
3._____
4._____
5._____

One thing I could do better: _____

How can I achieve it? _____

_____

NOTES

Day 5

DID I?

Eat healthy?
Yes   No

Eat when I wasn't hungry?
Yes   No

Work out?
Yes   No
If yes, what did I do?
_____

Walk/Run one mile?
Yes   No

Read 15 pages/chapters?
Yes   No
If yes, what did I read?
_____

Pray 15 minutes?
Yes   No

Eat fruit/vegetables?
Yes   No

Listen to a Christian Podcast?
Yes   No
If yes, what did I listen to?
_____

Rest without napping?
Yes   No

Five things I did good or like about myself today:

1. _____
2. _____
3. _____
4. _____
5. _____

One thing I could do better: _____

How can I achieve it? _____

_____

NOTES

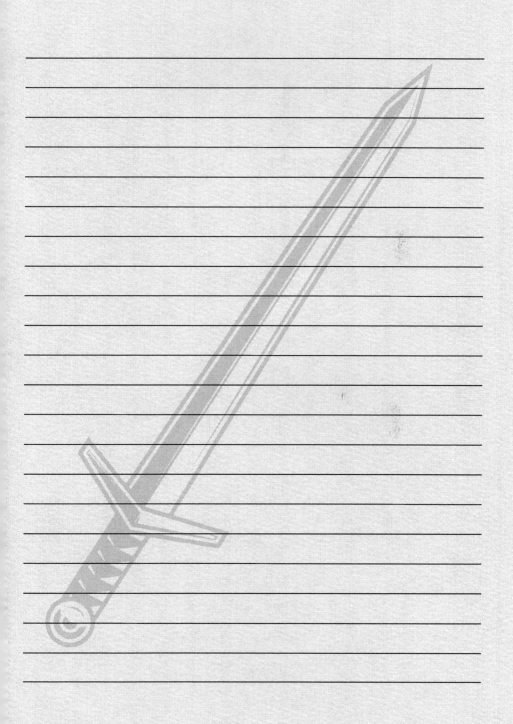

Day 6

DID I?

Eat healthy?
Yes   No

Eat when I wasn't hungry?
Yes   No

Work out?
Yes   No
If yes, what did I do?
_____

Walk/Run one mile?
Yes   No

Read 15 pages/chapters?
Yes   No
If yes, what did I read?
_____

Pray 15 minutes?
Yes   No

Eat fruit/vegetables?
Yes   No

Listen to a Christian Podcast?
Yes   No
If yes, what did I listen to?
_____

Rest without napping?
Yes   No

Five things I did good or like about myself today:

1. _____
2. _____
3. _____
4. _____
5. _____

One thing I could do better: _____

How can I achieve it? _____

_____

NOTES

Day 7

DID I?

Eat healthy?
Yes   No

Eat when I wasn't hungry?
Yes   No

Work out?
Yes   No
If yes, what did I do?
_____

Walk/Run one mile?
Yes   No

Read 15 pages/chapters?
Yes   No
If yes, what did I read?
_____

Pray 15 minutes?
Yes   No

Eat fruit/vegetables?
Yes   No

Listen to a Christian Podcast?
Yes   No
If yes, what did I listen to?
_____

Rest without napping?
Yes   No

Five things I did good or like about myself today:

1. _____
2. _____
3. _____
4. _____
5. _____

One thing I could do better: _____

How can I achieve it? _____
_____

NOTES

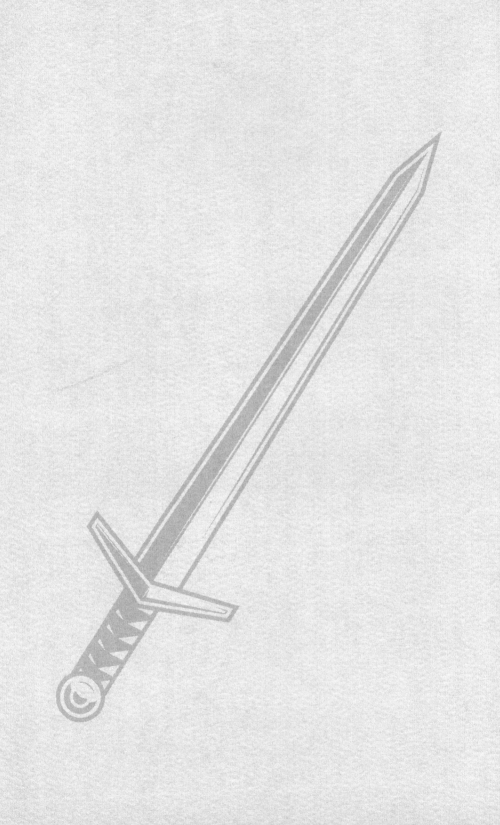

Made in the USA
Columbia, SC
25 June 2024

37346947R00098